Independent CMDA Exam Prep 2027–2028:

800 Practice Questions & Detailed Explanations for the Certified Medical Device Auditor Certification

Caldwell Abiodun

Author Introduction

In the highly regulated and rapidly evolving field of medical technology, the role of a Certified Medical Device Auditor (CMDA) is both critical and complex. Ensuring that medical device manufacturers meet stringent international standards requires not only technical expertise, but also a deep understanding of regulatory frameworks, quality management systems, and risk-based thinking. This study guide has been developed under the direction of a seasoned auditing professional, working in close collaboration with a dedicated team of quality specialists and regulatory experts, to support candidates preparing for the Certified Medical Device Auditor (CMDA) examination.

With extensive experience in auditing medical device organizations against globally recognized standards, the lead author brings a practical, real-world perspective to the material presented in this guide. Having conducted and overseen numerous first-, second-, and third-party audits, the author understands the nuanced expectations of certification bodies, regulatory authorities, and industry stakeholders. This expertise is complemented by a collaborative network of professionals specializing in quality management systems, risk management, design controls, supplier evaluation, and post-market surveillance—ensuring that every chapter reflects both technical accuracy and industry relevance.

The CMDA examination demands more than memorization of standards; it requires the ability to interpret requirements, assess compliance objectively, and apply auditing principles in complex operational environments. This guide is structured to build that competence systematically. Concepts are explained with clarity and depth, supported by scenario-based insights that mirror real audit situations. Emphasis is placed on ISO 13485 requirements, regulatory alignment, process-based auditing, corrective and preventive action (CAPA) systems, and the ethical responsibilities inherent in the auditing profession.

Throughout this resource, the focus remains firmly on candidate success. Each section is designed not only to reinforce foundational knowledge but also to sharpen critical thinking and decision-making skills essential for audit effectiveness. Practice-oriented explanations help bridge the gap between theory and application, empowering readers to approach the examination—and their professional responsibilities—with confidence.

This study guide reflects a commitment to advancing excellence within the medical device industry. By combining practical auditing experience with instructional precision, the author and contributing experts aim to equip aspiring Certified Medical Device Auditors with the competence, integrity, and insight required to uphold the highest standards of quality and patient safety.

Table of Content

Chapter 1: Auditing Fundamentals

The Purpose and Scope of Auditing

Auditing within the medical device industry serves as a structured, independent, and documented process for verifying compliance with established standards, regulations, and internal quality management requirements. The auditor's task is to determine whether systems, processes, and products conform to planned arrangements and to evaluate the effectiveness of implementation.

Audits are integral to maintaining control, ensuring continuous improvement, and protecting public health through verification of safety and efficacy across the device lifecycle. An audit is not merely a fault-finding activity but a **systematic evaluation of conformity and performance**.

The scope of a medical device audit often encompasses multiple regulatory and quality dimensions, such as adherence to **ISO 13485**, **21 CFR Part 820**, and relevant **Medical Device Single Audit Program (MDSAP)** criteria. Through this integrated scope, auditors ensure that organizations meet both the regulatory obligations and the operational goals of quality management.

Auditors must demonstrate independence, objectivity, and ethical integrity throughout the process. Their findings provide management with factual information to make informed decisions regarding corrective actions and system improvement.

Principles of Auditing

Auditing principles form the ethical and procedural foundation for credible audit execution. The core principles include **integrity**, **fair presentation**, **due professional care**, **confidentiality**, **independence**, and **evidence-based approach**.

- **Integrity** establishes trust and underpins the auditor's commitment to ethical conduct.
- **Fair presentation** requires that audit findings, conclusions, and reports accurately reflect observed facts.
- **Due professional care** ensures diligence and competence appropriate to the significance of the audit task.
- **Confidentiality** safeguards information obtained during the audit process.
- **Independence** ensures objectivity and impartial judgment.
- **Evidence-based approach** supports rational and reproducible conclusions derived from verifiable audit evidence.

These principles, adapted from **ISO 19011:2018**, form the ethical framework that guides professional auditing practice. When applied within medical device settings, they reinforce regulatory trust and ensure transparency in demonstrating compliance to authorities such as the FDA, EU Notified Bodies, or MDSAP regulatory partners.

Adherence to these principles also supports organizational credibility during third-party and regulatory audits, where the accuracy and impartiality of internal audits are often reviewed.

Roles and Responsibilities of the Auditor

A competent auditor possesses a combination of technical knowledge, auditing experience, and interpersonal skills. The auditor's role extends beyond documentation review—it encompasses the ability to interpret requirements, evaluate objective evidence, and communicate findings in a manner conducive to improvement.

The **lead auditor** bears primary responsibility for audit planning, resource allocation, team coordination, and communication with management. Supporting auditors may focus on specific areas, such as risk management, validation, or production controls, depending on their technical expertise.

Competence requirements for medical device auditors include knowledge of applicable standards, understanding of product realization processes, and awareness of risk management practices under ISO 14971. Auditors must remain alert to ethical obligations, avoiding conflicts of interest and maintaining professional skepticism.

Effective auditors balance technical precision with professional diplomacy. Communication must remain objective and factual, avoiding prescriptive or judgmental language. Reports should document both conformity and nonconformity in terms of evidence and applicable requirements.

Ultimately, auditors serve as agents of improvement, helping organizations identify weaknesses, confirm strengths, and maintain a state of continuous compliance. The credibility of audit outcomes depends entirely on the auditor's ability to act independently, evaluate evidence rigorously, and maintain professionalism throughout the audit lifecycle.

Audit Program Management

An audit program is a coordinated set of activities designed to plan, organize, and conduct audits according to defined objectives and schedules. Within the context of medical device quality systems, the audit program serves as a management tool to ensure that audits are conducted consistently and that findings contribute meaningfully to continuous improvement.

The program is typically established under the direction of senior management or the quality manager, reflecting both regulatory requirements and internal strategic priorities. For medical device organizations, the audit program must incorporate **risk-based planning**, ensuring that critical processes such as design control, production, validation, and post-market surveillance receive appropriate emphasis.

Audit program management involves defining the audit scope, frequency, methods, and responsibilities. Documentation of these elements provides traceability and consistency across audit cycles. In practice, an effective audit program integrates multiple layers of assessment—internal audits, supplier audits, and external regulatory audits—forming a comprehensive system for verifying compliance and driving improvement.

Regular management review of audit program performance ensures alignment with regulatory expectations under ISO 13485:2016 Clause 8.2.4 and FDA 21 CFR 820.22. Adjustments to the program are based on prior findings, risk analysis, and changes in organizational operations or regulatory requirements.

Audit Preparation

Audit preparation establishes the foundation for an efficient and effective audit process. Preparation begins with the **definition of audit objectives**, which determine the depth and scope of evaluation. Objectives may include verifying compliance with internal procedures, assessing effectiveness of quality system implementation, or confirming readiness for external inspection.

A formal **audit plan** outlines the processes to be audited, relevant standards and regulations, applicable documents, responsible personnel, and a detailed schedule. This plan must be reviewed and approved by the audit client (management) prior to execution.

Key preparatory activities include:

- Reviewing previous audit reports and corrective actions.
- Assessing changes in products, processes, or regulations since the last audit.
- Identifying applicable requirements (e.g., ISO 13485 clauses, 21 CFR 820 sections).
- Selecting and briefing the audit team based on competence and independence.
- Preparing audit checklists and evidence collection tools.

Audit preparation also involves logistical considerations such as scheduling, access to facilities, and document availability. The use of checklists, when appropriately designed, assists in maintaining focus and ensuring consistent evaluation, but auditors must avoid checklist dependency and instead apply judgment and flexibility to follow objective evidence wherever it leads.

Proper preparation ensures the audit proceeds smoothly, minimizes disruption, and increases the reliability of results. It also demonstrates professionalism and respect for the auditee, reinforcing the cooperative nature of auditing as an improvement process.

Audit Types and Classifications

Audits within the medical device sector can be categorized according to purpose, scope, and relationship between the auditor and the auditee. The principal classifications are **first-party (internal)**, **second-party (supplier)**, and **third-party (external or certification)** audits.

- **First-party audits** are conducted by or on behalf of the organization itself to verify conformity and identify opportunities for improvement. They form the core of ISO 13485 Clause 8.2.4 and FDA internal audit expectations.
- **Second-party audits** are performed by an organization on its suppliers or contractors to ensure compliance with contractual and regulatory requirements. Supplier audits are critical for verifying

control over purchased materials, outsourced processes, and external services that affect product quality.

- **Third-party audits** include certification or regulatory audits conducted by independent bodies such as Notified Bodies under the EU MDR or the FDA during inspections. These audits verify formal compliance and can influence market authorization or certification status.

Audits can also be distinguished by approach—**system audits**, **process audits**, and **product audits**. System audits evaluate the overall management system; process audits focus on the effectiveness and control of specific activities; and product audits confirm that finished devices meet defined specifications and labeling requirements.

The selection of audit type depends on objectives, regulatory drivers, and organizational priorities. Understanding these classifications enables auditors to adapt methodologies and reporting structures appropriately, ensuring that each audit yields meaningful insight into compliance and performance.

Audit Evidence

Audit evidence consists of verifiable information, records, and statements of fact gathered during an audit and used to determine the extent to which audit criteria are fulfilled. In medical device auditing, the evidence must be objective, traceable, and sufficient to support conclusions regarding compliance and system performance.

Evidence can be **qualitative or quantitative**, depending on the nature of the process evaluated. For example, calibration records, validation reports, and batch release data provide measurable evidence, while management interviews and procedural reviews offer qualitative insight.

The collection of audit evidence requires structured observation, inquiry, and document review. Auditors must ensure that evidence is representative, reliable, and obtained through appropriate sampling techniques. The degree of sampling depends on the audit scope, complexity, and risk level of the process under examination.

Documented evidence should directly link findings to specific requirements such as clauses of ISO 13485, sections of 21 CFR 820, or internal procedures. Each observation must be clearly referenced to maintain transparency and enable verification during subsequent reviews.

Audit evidence serves as the factual basis for findings and must withstand scrutiny from both the auditee and external regulators. Maintaining accuracy and neutrality in evidence collection reinforces the credibility of audit outcomes and ensures that recommendations for improvement are grounded in verifiable data.

Audit Findings and Classifications

Audit findings are the outcomes derived from evaluating audit evidence against the defined audit criteria. Findings may indicate **conformity**, **nonconformity**, or **opportunities for improvement**. Each must be documented in precise, factual, and traceable language.

A **nonconformity** represents failure to meet a requirement—whether derived from a regulatory clause, standard, or internal procedure. Nonconformities are generally classified according to severity:

- **Major Nonconformity:** A systemic or significant failure affecting compliance or product safety (e.g., lack of documented design validation).
- **Minor Nonconformity:** An isolated deviation not directly affecting product quality or safety (e.g., incomplete record signature).

Effective auditors distinguish between isolated errors and systemic weaknesses. Correct classification ensures that corrective actions are proportional and resources are allocated appropriately.

In addition to nonconformities, auditors may identify **observations**—noteworthy conditions that, while not direct violations, could lead to noncompliance if left unaddressed. **Opportunities for Improvement (OFIs)** are suggestions aimed at enhancing efficiency or robustness within the quality management system.

Each finding must be supported by corresponding evidence, explicitly linked to the requirement evaluated, and recorded in an audit log or checklist. Clear communication of findings during the closing meeting is essential to avoid misinterpretation and to promote constructive dialogue between auditor and auditee.

Audit Reporting and Follow-up

The audit report is the formal output of the audit process and serves as an official record of results, conclusions, and recommendations. It must be concise, accurate, and delivered in a timely manner to management. The report typically includes:

- Audit objectives, scope, and criteria.
- Identification of the audit team and participants.
- Summary of activities performed and evidence examined.
- Documented findings, including classification and applicable references.
- Conclusions regarding system conformity and effectiveness.

Follow-up actions are an integral part of the audit cycle. The auditor verifies that corrective and preventive actions (CAPA) have been implemented effectively and that they address the root cause of nonconformities. Verification may occur through documentation review, on-site reassessment, or targeted follow-up audits.

Timely closure of nonconformities and evidence-based verification of corrective actions demonstrate management's commitment to continual improvement and regulatory compliance.

Chapter I Summary

Auditing fundamentals establish the essential framework for all subsequent Chapters in the CMDA Body of Knowledge. The auditor's role, guided by ethical principles and professional competence, ensures that medical device organizations operate in alignment with international standards and regulatory requirements.

Mastery of this Chapter equips candidates to:

- Apply auditing principles with integrity and objectivity.
- Design, manage, and execute audit programs aligned with ISO 19011.
- Collect, evaluate, and report audit evidence effectively.
- Communicate findings and facilitate continual improvement.

Competent auditors contribute directly to regulatory confidence, product safety, and organizational excellence. The professional discipline cultivated here forms the cornerstone of all advanced auditing and compliance activities explored in the subsequent Chapters.

Chapter 2: Auditing and Inspection Processes

Audit Execution

The execution phase translates the audit plan into systematic action. It begins with verification of the audit's readiness, confirmation of logistical arrangements, and briefing of the audit team. During execution, auditors gather and evaluate evidence through interviews, observation, and document review, ensuring each activity directly supports the audit objectives and criteria.

Audit execution requires discipline and precision. The auditor's responsibility is to maintain alignment with the plan while exercising flexibility when new evidence or process deviations arise. Deviations from the audit plan must be justified, documented, and communicated to the lead auditor or audit client.

Auditors should maintain neutrality in tone and body language, fostering a professional atmosphere that encourages open communication. In medical device settings, audit execution often involves examination of controlled environments, validation records, calibration systems, and process controls associated with manufacturing, packaging, and labeling.

Documented notes, photographs (if permitted), and record identifiers are collected to support traceability of observations. Each data point should be verifiable and tied to specific quality system requirements, such as ISO 13485 clause references or CFR Part 820 subparts. Precision during execution ensures that the audit remains credible, reproducible, and defensible during regulatory scrutiny.

Conducting Opening and Closing Meetings

The **opening meeting** marks the formal start of the audit and establishes mutual understanding between the auditor and auditee. Its purpose is to confirm audit scope, objectives, timing, and responsibilities. A professional and structured opening meeting sets the tone for cooperation and transparency throughout the audit.

Key points covered in the opening meeting include:

- Introduction of audit team members and auditee representatives.
- Review of audit objectives, criteria, and methods.
- Confirmation of logistics, communication protocols, and safety considerations.
- Clarification of document access and confidentiality expectations.
- Opportunity for the auditee to raise questions or identify constraints.

Following the audit's completion, the **closing meeting** provides formal presentation of findings, conclusions, and next steps. The auditor summarizes results, identifies any nonconformities or observations, and verifies that the auditee clearly understands each issue. Findings must be presented factually, avoiding subjective or speculative language.

The closing meeting ensures transparency, gives the auditee an opportunity to clarify misunderstandings, and reinforces the principle of cooperative improvement. Both meetings are documented in the audit record, confirming procedural integrity and compliance with ISO 19011 guidance.

Sampling Techniques and Audit Evidence Sufficiency

Auditors rely on sampling because it is rarely feasible to examine every record or product. **Audit sampling** is a selective approach used to evaluate representative evidence that supports conclusions about overall system effectiveness.

Sampling methods are typically classified as **judgmental** or **statistical**:

- **Judgmental (non-statistical) sampling** depends on the auditor's expertise and experience to select areas of highest risk or significance. This approach is common in regulatory audits where specific compliance risks are known or anticipated.
- **Statistical sampling** applies mathematical techniques to determine sample size and selection, offering measurable confidence levels. It is often used in process validation, inspection data review, or when evaluating large data sets.

The adequacy of sampling depends on factors such as process complexity, past performance, and criticality of the operation. In auditing medical device processes, auditors should focus sampling on records that impact product quality and patient safety—such as complaint files, CAPA documentation, sterilization records, and supplier evaluations.

Auditors must document their rationale for sampling and ensure that evidence collected is sufficient, appropriate, and representative. Inadequate or biased sampling undermines the reliability of findings and may lead to incorrect conclusions.

Sound sampling practices uphold the integrity of the audit process and demonstrate to regulators that evaluations are performed with professional rigor and due diligence.

Interviewing Techniques

Interviewing is a principal method for gathering audit evidence and validating process understanding. A skilled auditor must conduct interviews that elicit clear, objective information without leading the respondent or implying conclusions.

The purpose of the audit interview is to verify that personnel understand their responsibilities, apply procedures correctly, and maintain control over regulated activities. Questions should be open-ended, encouraging explanation rather than simple affirmation. For example, instead of asking, "Do you follow this procedure?" the auditor may ask, "Can you describe how you perform this process and how you verify its completion?"

Effective interviewers listen attentively, observe body language, and cross-check verbal responses with documented evidence or on-site observations. Consistency between documentation and practice is a strong indicator of system control. Discrepancies, however, should be explored factually rather than confrontationally, maintaining a professional and cooperative tone.

Auditors must also respect confidentiality and avoid questioning employees about topics outside their responsibility. Interview summaries should be recorded in audit notes, including the role of the interviewee, the process discussed, and supporting evidence reviewed. Interviews, when conducted systematically, validate the competence of personnel and the integrity of the quality management system.

Traceability and Audit Trails

Traceability is fundamental to medical device quality assurance and a key focus during audits. It ensures that every product, process, and document can be traced backward and forward through all stages of design, manufacturing, distribution, and post-market surveillance.

An **audit trail** represents the documented linkage between evidence sources, such as procedures, records, and product identifiers. Traceability enables auditors to follow the logical flow from input to output, confirming that each step meets defined requirements.

Typical traceability chains examined during audits include:

- Design inputs → design outputs → verification/validation → production specifications.
- Component identification → batch or lot tracking → device history records → distribution logs.
- Complaint records → CAPA actions → verification of effectiveness.

Regulatory frameworks such as ISO 13485:2016 (Clause 7.5.9.2) and FDA 21 CFR 820.65 mandate that traceability be maintained for devices where safety and performance are critical. Effective audit trails confirm that organizations can identify affected devices during recalls, field actions, or investigations.

Auditors should evaluate the completeness, accuracy, and accessibility of traceability records. Missing links, inconsistent data, or unverified transfers between departments signal potential nonconformities. Strong traceability systems not only ensure compliance but also enhance organizational control and confidence in product integrity.

Integration of Inspection Processes

Inspection processes represent the operational complement to auditing within the medical device quality framework. While auditing assesses system effectiveness, **inspection** evaluates tangible product and process conformity. Integration of these two disciplines strengthens both verification and preventive control.

Auditors frequently examine inspection data to validate that monitoring activities are effective. Key elements include inspection plans, acceptance criteria, sampling procedures, and documentation of results. The auditor assesses whether inspection outcomes are analyzed for trends and whether corrective actions are initiated when acceptance limits are exceeded.

Integration between audit and inspection processes is achieved when inspection results feed back into the audit program, influencing risk assessment, audit scheduling, and focus areas. This closed-loop system supports continual improvement by aligning operational monitoring with strategic oversight.

In regulatory terms, the inspection process must conform to requirements such as ISO 13485 Clause 8.2.6 ("Monitoring and Measurement of Product") and FDA 21 CFR 820.80 ("Receiving, In-Process, and Finished Device Acceptance"). These clauses require objective evidence that inspection activities ensure product safety and conformity.

By validating inspection systems during audits, organizations demonstrate proactive control over process outcomes and readiness for external regulatory inspection. This integration embodies the principle of total quality assurance—where every function supports consistent compliance and patient safety.

Audit Reporting

Audit reporting within the medical device industry requires precision, objectivity, and timeliness. The audit report documents all relevant observations, evidence, and conclusions derived from the audit process. It serves as the formal communication tool between the auditor, auditee, and management, ensuring accountability and traceability of findings.

A well-structured report typically includes:

1. **Administrative details:** audit title, scope, date, team members, and auditee identification.
2. **Audit objectives and criteria:** reference to applicable standards and regulations such as ISO 13485, 21 CFR 820, and relevant internal procedures.
3. **Summary of activities:** description of processes reviewed, interviews conducted, and evidence examined.
4. **Findings:** categorized as conformities, nonconformities, observations, or opportunities for improvement.
5. **Conclusions and recommendations:** overall evaluation of system effectiveness and proposed actions.

Reports should be written in concise, factual language free from opinion or conjecture. Each finding must be substantiated by clear evidence and referenced to a specific requirement. Management should receive the report promptly after the audit, allowing timely corrective action planning.

Audit reporting demonstrates transparency and is often reviewed during external inspections as evidence of a functioning quality management system. Proper documentation enhances confidence in both internal and third-party audits, reinforcing organizational integrity and compliance.

Regulatory Inspection Readiness

Regulatory inspections conducted by authorities such as the U.S. Food and Drug Administration (FDA) or European Union Notified Bodies are formal evaluations of a company's compliance with applicable laws and regulations. Preparation for these inspections shares many characteristics with audit readiness but requires heightened attention to documentation accuracy, personnel competence, and immediate availability of records.

Inspection readiness is an ongoing process, not a short-term event. Organizations must maintain systems that ensure continuous compliance, allowing them to demonstrate control at any time. Elements critical to readiness include:

- Comprehensive and current documentation of quality system procedures and records.
- Trained staff who can clearly explain their processes and responsibilities.
- Rapid retrieval systems for records such as Device History Files, CAPA logs, and complaint data.
- Evidence of management review, risk management, and post-market surveillance activities.

Internal audits act as the first line of defense in maintaining inspection readiness. They identify and correct deficiencies before regulatory authorities do. Auditors play a key role in evaluating preparedness through simulated inspection exercises, also known as "mock inspections," which mirror the depth and rigor of actual regulatory reviews.

Sustained readiness reflects a culture of quality and demonstrates that compliance is integrated into daily operations, not merely a response to oversight.

Chapter II Summary

Auditing and inspection processes together form the operational backbone of medical device compliance assurance. Through structured execution, disciplined communication, and factual reporting, auditors validate that systems operate as intended and that evidence supports compliance with regulatory and quality requirements.

By mastering this Chapter, CMDA candidates will be able to:

- Conduct audits with professional rigor and evidence-based judgment.
- Manage opening and closing meetings to foster transparent communication.
- Apply effective sampling and interviewing techniques to obtain representative evidence.
- Evaluate traceability, inspection records, and process control for conformity.
- Demonstrate inspection readiness aligned with global regulatory expectations.

Successful auditors integrate auditing and inspection as complementary functions—one providing assurance of system integrity, the other confirming product and process conformity. Together they enable medical device organizations to maintain continuous compliance, ensure patient safety, and uphold regulatory confidence.

Chapter 3: Medical Device Quality Management System Requirements

Regulatory Foundations

The regulatory framework governing medical devices establishes the foundation for quality management systems worldwide. Its primary objective is to ensure that medical devices are consistently designed, manufactured, and distributed in a manner that guarantees their safety and effectiveness.

The **U.S. Food and Drug Administration (FDA)** and the **International Organization for Standardization (ISO)** serve as principal authorities in defining QMS expectations. In the United States, **21 CFR Part 820**, known as the **Quality System Regulation (QSR)**, outlines the legal requirements manufacturers must follow. Internationally, **ISO 13485:2016** provides a harmonized standard applicable to organizations engaged in any aspect of the medical device life cycle, from design to post-market activities.

Together, these frameworks define the systematic controls necessary for product realization, risk management, and regulatory compliance. They align conceptually under the principles of documentation control, management responsibility, resource management, product realization, and measurement, analysis, and improvement.

While compliance with ISO 13485 facilitates global market access through harmonization with the Medical Device Single Audit Program (MDSAP), adherence to 21 CFR Part 820 remains mandatory for products marketed in the United States. The forthcoming **Quality Management System Regulation (QMSR)** initiative seeks to further align FDA requirements with ISO 13485, ensuring consistency and reducing redundancy across jurisdictions.

Structure of ISO 13485:2016

ISO 13485 establishes a structured and process-based approach to quality management tailored specifically for the medical device industry. It defines requirements for a QMS where an organization must demonstrate its ability to provide medical devices and related services that consistently meet customer and regulatory requirements.

The standard is organized into the following key clauses:

1. **Clause 4 – Quality Management System:** General requirements and documentation control, including the maintenance of a quality manual and control of records.
2. **Clause 5 – Management Responsibility:** Leadership commitment, customer focus, quality policy, and management review processes.
3. **Clause 6 – Resource Management:** Competence, infrastructure, and work environment necessary for process control.
4. **Clause 7 – Product Realization:** Planning, design, purchasing, production, and service provision—all governed by risk management and validation principles.
5. **Clause 8 – Measurement, Analysis, and Improvement:** Monitoring processes, internal audits, nonconformity control, and continual improvement.

ISO 13485 differs from ISO 9001 by emphasizing regulatory compliance, risk management, and sterile device control over customer satisfaction metrics. The standard requires documented evidence of process validation, cleanliness, traceability, and the effectiveness of corrective and preventive actions.

For auditors, familiarity with the structure and intent of ISO 13485 is essential. Each clause represents a potential audit trail and provides a basis for evaluating conformity between documented processes and actual practices.

FDA 21 CFR Part 820: Quality System Regulation

The FDA's Quality System Regulation (QSR), codified under **Title 21 of the Code of Federal Regulations Part 820**, establishes the minimum requirements for the design, manufacture, packaging, labeling, storage, installation, and servicing of finished medical devices intended for human use.

The QSR is structured similarly to ISO 13485 but framed in regulatory language that mandates compliance. Key subparts include:

- **Subpart B – Quality System Requirements:** Management responsibility, quality planning, and personnel training.
- **Subpart C – Design Controls:** Procedures for design input, output, review, verification, validation, transfer, and change management.
- **Subpart G – Production and Process Controls:** Validation, environmental controls, equipment maintenance, and process monitoring.
- **Subpart H – Acceptance Activities:** Receiving, in-process, and final inspections ensuring product conformity.
- **Subpart J – Corrective and Preventive Actions (CAPA):** Mechanisms to identify and eliminate causes of nonconformities.
- **Subpart M – Records:** Device history, device master records, and complaint handling documentation.

The QSR emphasizes the establishment of procedures and documentation that demonstrate consistent compliance. Auditors must evaluate both the existence and effectiveness of these systems, ensuring they are implemented and maintained as written.

Alignment between ISO 13485 and 21 CFR 820 enables organizations to maintain a unified QMS framework that satisfies both domestic and international requirements, reducing duplication and facilitating regulatory audits.

Design and Development Controls

Design and development controls represent the central framework through which medical devices are conceptualized, designed, verified, validated, and transferred into production. These controls ensure that design outputs meet intended use requirements, user needs, and applicable regulatory expectations.

Under **ISO 13485 Clause 7.3** and **21 CFR 820.30**, manufacturers must establish and maintain procedures to control the design of devices to ensure that specified design requirements are met. The process begins with **design planning**, where stages, responsibilities, and review mechanisms are defined.

- **Design Inputs** must be clearly documented and include functional, performance, regulatory, and user requirements.
- **Design Outputs** translate these inputs into tangible specifications such as drawings, formulations, and manufacturing instructions.
- **Design Review** activities assess progress and verify that the design remains aligned with its objectives.
- **Design Verification** confirms that outputs meet inputs through testing and analysis.
- **Design Validation** ensures that the final product fulfills user and clinical needs under actual or simulated conditions of use.
- **Design Transfer** establishes that production capabilities can reliably replicate the validated design.
- **Design Changes** must be controlled and documented to prevent unintended impact on performance or safety.

Auditors must verify that these elements are fully traceable, with documented linkages among inputs, outputs, verification, and validation records. A lack of design traceability or incomplete validation constitutes a significant nonconformity under both ISO and FDA frameworks.

Risk Management Integration

Risk management is a regulatory expectation that spans the entire product life cycle. The principles are codified in **ISO 14971:2019**, which requires that manufacturers identify, evaluate, control, and monitor risks associated with medical devices. ISO 13485 integrates these principles directly into design and product realization activities.

The risk management process involves:

1. **Risk Analysis** – Identifying hazards related to device characteristics and use conditions.
2. **Risk Evaluation** – Determining the probability of occurrence and severity of harm.
3. **Risk Control** – Implementing measures to reduce risk to an acceptable level through design modifications, protective measures, or labeling.
4. **Residual Risk Evaluation** – Ensuring remaining risks are acceptable when weighed against benefits.
5. **Risk Review** – Maintaining an updated risk management file throughout post-market activities.

Auditors should assess whether risk management is embedded in organizational processes and not treated as a standalone exercise. Evidence may include risk management plans, FMEA (Failure Mode and Effects Analysis) records, and linkage between risk control measures and verification or validation outcomes.

Regulatory authorities expect that manufacturers maintain active risk management files for every product. Incomplete or outdated files are indicators of systemic weakness. Auditors should confirm that risk-based thinking informs decision-making, process control, and post-market surveillance activities, demonstrating alignment with ISO 13485 and global expectations under the Medical Device Regulation (MDR).

Process Validation Activities

Process validation provides documented assurance that manufacturing processes consistently produce products meeting predetermined specifications and quality attributes. Validation is particularly critical for processes where output cannot be fully verified by subsequent inspection or testing, such as sterilization, sealing, or molding.

The regulatory basis for process validation is found in **ISO 13485 Clause 7.5.6** and **FDA 21 CFR 820.75**. Both require manufacturers to establish protocols defining validation methodology, acceptance criteria, equipment qualification, and documentation requirements.

Key stages of validation include:

- **Installation Qualification (IQ):** Verification that equipment is installed according to specifications.
- **Operational Qualification (OQ):** Demonstration that the process operates within defined limits and tolerances.
- **Performance Qualification (PQ):** Confirmation that the process consistently produces output meeting quality criteria under normal conditions.

Auditors evaluate validation files to verify that protocols are approved before execution, that deviations are documented and justified, and that revalidation occurs after significant process or equipment changes.

Inadequate validation can compromise device quality and patient safety, leading to regulatory action. Effective validation programs demonstrate scientific rigor, traceability, and control, thereby ensuring that device manufacturing remains both compliant and reliable throughout the product life cycle.

Supplier Management and Purchasing Controls

Supplier management forms a crucial component of a compliant medical device quality system. Because manufacturers frequently rely on external suppliers for materials, components, and services, regulatory frameworks demand evidence that all purchased items conform to specified requirements.

ISO 13485 Clause 7.4 and **FDA 21 CFR 820.50** require that organizations evaluate and select suppliers based on their ability to meet established specifications. This process must be documented through procedures that define supplier qualification, monitoring, and re-evaluation criteria.

Key elements include:

- **Supplier Evaluation and Approval:** Based on audits, quality performance history, and capability assessments.
- **Purchasing Data Control:** Purchase orders must clearly describe requirements, including material specifications, acceptance criteria, and reference to applicable regulations or standards.
- **Supplier Monitoring:** Periodic review of supplier performance using metrics such as on-time delivery, defect rates, and corrective action responsiveness.
- **Supplier Audits:** Conducted as part of a risk-based strategy to verify ongoing compliance.

Auditors should verify that supplier files contain qualification evidence, contracts or quality agreements, and records of performance reviews. A lack of supplier oversight poses a significant compliance risk, as suppliers directly influence the integrity of finished devices. Robust supplier management reflects an organization's control over its entire supply chain and ensures regulatory confidence in product conformity.

Corrective and Preventive Action (CAPA) Systems

The CAPA system serves as the backbone of continuous improvement and regulatory compliance. It provides the formal mechanism for identifying, investigating, and eliminating the causes of actual and potential nonconformities.

Both **ISO 13485 Clause 8.5.2–8.5.3** and **FDA 21 CFR 820.100** require organizations to establish procedures for CAPA implementation. A compliant CAPA system typically includes:

1. **Problem Identification:** Through nonconformity reports, complaints, audits, or trend analysis.
2. **Root Cause Analysis:** Systematic evaluation using tools such as the 5 Whys or Ishikawa diagrams.
3. **Action Planning:** Determination of corrective or preventive measures appropriate to the problem's significance.
4. **Implementation:** Execution of planned actions with assigned responsibilities and due dates.
5. **Verification of Effectiveness:** Review to confirm that implemented actions prevent recurrence or occurrence.
6. **Documentation and Review:** Maintaining records demonstrating traceability, closure, and management oversight.

Auditors should examine CAPA records for completeness, timeliness, and evidence of data-driven analysis. Ineffective CAPA systems—such as those focused only on symptoms or lacking verification—are among the most common findings in FDA warning letters.

A robust CAPA process transforms compliance into proactive quality improvement. By addressing systemic issues rather than isolated incidents, it enhances reliability, reduces risk, and sustains regulatory confidence.

Management Review

Management review provides the formal mechanism through which executive leadership evaluates the overall performance and suitability of the quality management system. It is both a regulatory requirement and a strategic practice, ensuring that senior management remains accountable for compliance and continuous improvement.

ISO 13485 Clause 5.6 and **21 CFR 820.20(c)** require that management reviews occur at planned intervals and are supported by documented evidence. These reviews must address:

- Audit results and corrective actions.
- Customer feedback and complaints.
- Process performance and product conformity.
- Resource needs, training, and infrastructure adequacy.
- Opportunities for improvement and changes affecting the QMS.

Meeting records must include inputs, outputs, and decisions. Outputs often involve actions related to quality objectives, process improvement, and allocation of resources.

Auditors should assess whether management reviews are timely, comprehensive, and result in tangible outcomes. Reviews that occur merely as procedural formality, without analysis or follow-up, fail to demonstrate effective management control.

Effective management review links organizational strategy with regulatory compliance, ensuring that quality remains an integral component of business performance. This commitment from leadership reinforces a culture of accountability, compliance, and continual improvement throughout the organization.

Documentation and Record Control

Documentation control ensures that all quality management system (QMS) documents are current, accurate, and readily accessible to authorized personnel. Within medical device organizations, documentation serves as the primary means of demonstrating compliance with regulatory requirements and effective system operation.

ISO 13485 Clause 4.2.4 and **FDA 21 CFR 820.40** establish strict expectations for document control. Procedures must define methods for document approval, distribution, revision, and retention. Controlled documents—such as procedures, work instructions, forms, and quality manuals—must be reviewed and approved prior to issue and updated when necessary to reflect process or regulatory changes.

Auditors should confirm that obsolete documents are promptly removed from points of use and that revision histories clearly record the nature of and reason for changes. Electronic document control systems, when utilized, must maintain audit trails showing authorship, approval, and modification dates.

In addition, document control extends to external standards, customer specifications, and supplier documentation used in product realization. Uncontrolled or outdated references can result in nonconformities during both internal and regulatory audits.

Document control underpins all other QMS processes; without it, the traceability and reliability of compliance evidence cannot be assured.

Recordkeeping and Data Integrity

Records serve as objective evidence that activities have been performed as required and that quality objectives have been achieved. They include test results, training records, production data, validation files, and complaint investigations. **ISO 13485 Clause 4.2.5** and **FDA 21 CFR 820.180** specify that records must be legible, readily identifiable, retrievable, and protected from damage or loss.

Electronic recordkeeping must also comply with **21 CFR Part 11**, which governs electronic records and signatures. Systems must incorporate access controls, audit trails, and validation demonstrating reliability and security.

Auditors evaluate records not merely for presence but for completeness, accuracy, and authenticity. Discrepancies between recorded and actual practices are strong indicators of procedural weakness. For instance, missing data entries, unauthorized changes, or inconsistent timestamps may signal lapses in data integrity.

Best practices include routine record review, periodic backups, and restricted access based on user roles. Training in documentation accuracy and data handling forms part of overall compliance culture. Records that are traceable and verifiable serve as the backbone of any successful audit or regulatory inspection, evidencing both conformity and accountability.

Chapter III Summary

Medical device quality management systems provide the structural and procedural backbone for regulatory compliance and product assurance. Through disciplined application of ISO 13485 and 21 CFR 820 requirements, organizations establish processes that ensure design integrity, process control, and continual improvement.

Upon completing this Chapter, CMDA candidates should be able to:

- Interpret the structure and interrelationship of ISO 13485 and 21 CFR 820.
- Evaluate design and development controls for adequacy, traceability, and validation.
- Verify integration of risk management, supplier oversight, and CAPA activities.
- Assess documentation and recordkeeping systems for control, accuracy, and security.
- Confirm management review effectiveness and leadership accountability.

An auditor proficient in QMS requirements transcends procedural evaluation to assess system maturity, data integrity, and organizational culture. This competence enables a holistic approach to compliance assurance and prepares auditors to engage confidently with global regulatory authorities.

Chapter III forms the bridge between auditing methodology and technical knowledge—setting the stage for evaluation of product-specific processes in the following Chapter.

Download Audio file and flashcards

Chapter 4: Technical Medical Device Knowledge

Product Lifecycle Overview

The medical device product lifecycle encompasses every stage from concept development through post-market monitoring. Each phase introduces distinct quality and regulatory requirements that must be understood and controlled. Auditors must be able to evaluate whether processes within each stage comply with both ISO and FDA expectations.

The lifecycle begins with **concept and feasibility**, where user needs, clinical requirements, and market analyses are translated into preliminary design inputs. The **design and development** stage formalizes those inputs, establishing specifications, prototypes, and risk management frameworks.

Once validated, the **design transfer** phase ensures that manufacturing processes, instructions, and inspection criteria can reliably reproduce the intended design. The **production and distribution** phase focuses on maintaining process control, ensuring that devices consistently meet defined specifications. Finally, the **post-market** phase—comprising complaint handling, vigilance, and field performance monitoring—closes the lifecycle loop through continuous feedback and improvement.

Auditors reviewing lifecycle management must verify the presence of defined interfaces among departments and confirm that handoffs between phases are documented and reviewed. Effective lifecycle control ensures traceability, mitigates risk, and supports long-term compliance across global markets.

Design Transfer and Production Readiness

Design transfer marks the critical transition between product development and manufacturing. Its objective is to ensure that design outputs—drawings, materials, software, and procedures—are accurately and completely translated into production specifications.

ISO 13485 Clause 7.3.8 and **21 CFR 820.30(h)** require documented procedures for transferring design to production. Auditors must confirm that these procedures define responsibilities, review mechanisms, and acceptance criteria for readiness.

Key audit checkpoints include:

- Verification that all design documents are approved and under version control before transfer.
- Confirmation that manufacturing equipment, software, and environmental controls are validated for their intended purpose.
- Review of training records demonstrating operator competency on new or modified processes.
- Evaluation of pilot runs or first-article inspections verifying that production processes meet specifications.

Deficiencies in design transfer often result in process variability and product nonconformities. Therefore, auditors must ensure that the transition from design to production is both systematic and evidence-based, minimizing the risk of uncontrolled deviations.

Effective design transfer reflects organizational maturity and readiness for full-scale production, bridging engineering intent with consistent operational execution.

Manufacturing Process Controls

Manufacturing process control is essential to ensuring product quality and compliance throughout routine production. These controls include methods, measurements, and monitoring activities that maintain consistency and detect deviation before it affects finished device quality.

Under **ISO 13485 Clause 7.5** and **FDA 21 CFR 820.70**, manufacturers are required to develop and implement documented procedures that define process parameters, equipment maintenance, environmental conditions, and personnel training.

Critical process control components include:

- **Process Parameters:** Defined and validated to ensure repeatability and reproducibility.
- **Equipment Calibration and Maintenance:** Verified through calibration schedules and maintenance logs.
- **Environmental Control:** Especially for sterile or cleanroom operations, including monitoring of temperature, humidity, and particulate levels.
- **In-Process Inspection and Monitoring:** Ensures ongoing verification of product characteristics.

Auditors should trace records to confirm adherence to process specifications and examine trend data for variation that may indicate control weakness. Deviations must be properly documented, investigated, and resolved through CAPA or revalidation activities.

A well-controlled manufacturing environment reflects adherence to regulatory principles of quality assurance—ensuring that every device produced is safe, effective, and consistent with its intended design.

Sterilization and Packaging Validation

Sterilization is a critical process in the manufacture of many medical devices, ensuring that products are free from viable microorganisms before reaching the end user. Because sterility cannot be verified by inspection alone, validation of sterilization processes is a regulatory requirement.

ISO 13485 Clause 7.5.7 and **FDA 21 CFR 820.75** require that sterilization processes—such as ethylene oxide (EtO), gamma irradiation, or steam sterilization—be validated before use and periodically revalidated. The validation must demonstrate that the process consistently achieves the specified sterility assurance level (SAL), typically 10^{-6} for sterile devices.

Key validation steps include:

- **Installation and Qualification:** Verifying sterilizer functionality and calibration.
- **Cycle Development and Validation:** Establishing parameters for time, temperature, humidity, and gas concentration (if applicable).

- **Microbiological Testing:** Determining bioburden, performing biological indicator studies, and confirming SAL achievement.
- **Revalidation:** Conducted after equipment modifications, process changes, or extended inactivity.

Packaging validation complements sterilization by confirming that sterile barriers maintain integrity throughout handling, transport, and storage. **ISO 11607** provides global guidance on packaging validation, including seal strength, material compatibility, and accelerated aging studies.

Auditors should verify that sterilization and packaging validations are documented, approved, and traceable to product specifications. Any deviation or failure to perform timely revalidation represents a serious nonconformity due to potential impact on patient safety.

Environmental Control Systems

Environmental control is essential to maintaining product quality, particularly for sterile and sensitive medical devices. Cleanroom environments must be designed, validated, and monitored to prevent contamination and maintain controlled conditions.

ISO 14644 and **ISO 13485 Clause 6.4** establish requirements for cleanroom classification, environmental monitoring, and maintenance. The FDA further enforces these controls under **21 CFR 820.70(c)**, which mandates that manufacturing areas be adequately controlled to prevent contamination or mix-ups.

Environmental control systems typically include:

- **Air Handling and Filtration Systems:** HEPA-filtered air maintaining specified particulate and microbial limits.
- **Temperature and Humidity Monitoring:** Continuous systems with alarm thresholds and data recording.
- **Personnel Gowning and Hygiene:** Procedures ensuring controlled entry and minimizing contamination risks.
- **Cleaning and Sanitization Protocols:** Validated to demonstrate microbial reduction effectiveness.

Auditors should review calibration records, environmental data logs, and deviation reports. Trending of environmental results helps identify deterioration in control and allows early corrective action.

Failure to maintain environmental control may result in compromised device quality, product recalls, and regulatory enforcement actions. An effective environmental control system demonstrates the organization's commitment to product safety and regulatory compliance.

Cleanroom Management and Contamination Control

Cleanroom management extends beyond facility design to encompass operational discipline, personnel behavior, and continuous monitoring. Auditors must verify that management systems ensure compliance with defined cleanroom classifications and operational parameters.

Critical aspects of cleanroom management include:

- **Personnel Training:** Employees must understand gowning procedures, contamination risks, and aseptic techniques.
- **Material Flow Control:** Segregation of sterile and non-sterile items, with unidirectional flow to prevent cross-contamination.
- **Monitoring and Trending:** Routine particulate and microbial testing, surface sampling, and air quality assessments.
- **Maintenance and Calibration:** Timely servicing of HVAC systems, pressure differentials, and filtration systems.
- **Change Control:** Documented review of modifications that may affect environmental performance.

Auditors evaluate whether records demonstrate consistent adherence to cleanroom procedures, including gown integrity checks, cleaning logs, and deviation handling. Cross-referencing of environmental results with production data helps identify correlations between control fluctuations and potential product quality issues.

Effective cleanroom management reflects an organization's operational maturity. It ensures that high-risk manufacturing environments remain stable and compliant—safeguarding device integrity and ultimately protecting patient health.

Post-Market Surveillance

Post-market surveillance (PMS) is the systematic process of collecting and analyzing information on the performance of medical devices once they are placed on the market. It provides essential feedback to ensure ongoing compliance, detect emerging risks, and maintain product safety throughout the device's life cycle.

ISO 13485 Clause 8.2.1 and regional regulations such as the **European Union Medical Device Regulation (MDR) Article 83** mandate that manufacturers establish and maintain PMS systems. Similarly, **FDA 21 CFR 820.198** requires procedures for complaint handling and trend analysis, forming part of a broader vigilance system.

A comprehensive PMS program includes:

- **Data Collection:** Information gathered from complaints, service reports, returned products, clinical evaluations, and field actions.
- **Trend Analysis:** Identification of recurring issues or deviations using statistical methods.
- **Risk Reevaluation:** Updating of risk management files when new data suggests increased risk.
- **Corrective Actions:** Initiation of CAPA, recalls, or labeling changes as necessary.

Auditors should verify that PMS processes are active, documented, and integrated with risk management and CAPA systems. Evidence of regular analysis and management review confirms compliance and organizational awareness.

Failure to conduct effective PMS can result in delayed identification of safety issues and potential regulatory action. A mature PMS system reflects a proactive culture that values patient safety as a continuous obligation rather than a post-market formality.

Complaint Handling

Complaint handling is a cornerstone of post-market quality assurance. It ensures that feedback regarding product performance, defects, or adverse events is captured, analyzed, and resolved appropriately.

ISO 13485 Clause 8.2.2 and **FDA 21 CFR 820.198** stipulate that manufacturers establish procedures for receiving, evaluating, and investigating complaints. Each complaint must be documented, evaluated for regulatory reporting requirements, and linked to risk management and CAPA systems.

Critical elements of an effective complaint handling process include:

- **Complaint Intake:** Defined channels for receiving information from customers, clinicians, or distributors.
- **Evaluation and Investigation:** Assessment of device history, lot traceability, and root cause determination.
- **Medical Device Reporting (MDR):** Timely submission of adverse event reports to authorities when required.
- **Trend Analysis:** Identification of recurring problems or systemic issues.
- **Feedback Loop:** Communication of findings to design, manufacturing, and management teams for corrective action.

Auditors should ensure complaint files contain sufficient evidence of evaluation, investigation outcomes, and closure justification. Inadequate documentation or lack of investigation is a critical nonconformity under both ISO and FDA frameworks.

Proper complaint management not only fulfills regulatory expectations but also provides valuable insight into real-world device performance, supporting continuous improvement and patient protection.

Chapter IV Summary

Technical knowledge of medical devices is essential for auditors to assess compliance effectively and identify risks specific to design, production, and post-market processes. Mastery of this Chapter ensures that auditors can evaluate the full product life cycle—from conception to field performance—with both technical accuracy and regulatory awareness.

CMDA candidates completing this Chapter should be able to:

- Interpret the interdependence between design, manufacturing, and post-market controls.
- Evaluate sterilization, packaging, and environmental systems for validation and maintenance.
- Verify the effectiveness of post-market surveillance and complaint-handling systems.
- Recognize potential risks arising from inadequate technical documentation or process validation.

Technical insight empowers auditors to move beyond procedural compliance and focus on the real-world performance and safety of medical devices. This knowledge fosters credibility with regulatory authorities and positions the auditor as a critical partner in ensuring public health protection and organizational excellence.

Chapter 5: Quality Tools and Techniques

Data Analysis for Quality Improvement

Data analysis enables auditors and quality professionals to identify trends, verify process performance, and support evidence-based decisions. Within the medical device industry, data-driven analysis forms the backbone of risk mitigation, continuous improvement, and regulatory compliance.

ISO 13485 Clause 8.4 and **21 CFR 820.100(a)(1)** require organizations to collect and analyze data from various sources—such as nonconformities, complaints, audit results, and process monitoring—to determine where improvements are necessary.

Effective data analysis involves:

- **Data Collection:** Ensuring accuracy, completeness, and relevance of input data.
- **Data Stratification:** Grouping data by source, process, or product type for clarity.
- **Trend Identification:** Detecting recurring patterns or deviations from control limits.
- **Actionable Interpretation:** Linking analysis to CAPA, management review, or risk assessment activities.

Common analytical tools include Pareto charts, run charts, control charts, and histograms. These visual methods simplify complex data sets, allowing users to focus on the most significant factors affecting quality.

Auditors assess whether data analysis processes are systematic, documented, and utilized in decision-making. A strong analytical culture ensures that quality management remains proactive rather than reactive.

Statistical Process Control (SPC)

Statistical Process Control (SPC) is a key technique for monitoring process behavior and maintaining product consistency. It relies on statistical methods to detect variation, identify special causes, and ensure that processes remain stable and capable.

Under regulatory expectations such as **ISO 13485 Clause 8.2.5** and **FDA 21 CFR 820.250**, manufacturers must validate and monitor processes using statistical techniques appropriate to the data collected.

SPC tools include:

- **Control Charts:** Used to track process performance over time, identifying trends or out-of-control conditions.
- **Process Capability Indices (Cp, Cpk):** Quantify how well a process meets specification limits.
- **Histogram Analysis:** Reveals distribution characteristics and variation spread.
- **Trend Analysis:** Detects shifts or drifts that may signal loss of control.

Auditors should confirm that SPC methods are applied to critical parameters, particularly in processes affecting device safety or performance. They should also verify that personnel interpreting SPC results are properly trained and that actions are documented when control limits are exceeded.

Effective SPC provides early warning of potential nonconformities, reduces process variability, and enhances confidence in product reliability—key attributes under both ISO and FDA regulatory oversight.

Root Cause Analysis (RCA) Methods

Root cause analysis (RCA) is the disciplined process of identifying the fundamental origin of a problem rather than its symptoms. It underpins both corrective and preventive action activities and ensures that issues are eliminated permanently rather than temporarily mitigated.

Common RCA techniques include:

- **The 5 Whys Method:** Sequential questioning to trace problems to their underlying cause.
- **Fishbone (Ishikawa) Diagram:** Categorizes potential causes into groups such as methods, materials, manpower, machines, and environment.
- **Failure Mode and Effects Analysis (FMEA):** Evaluates potential failure points, their consequences, and associated risk priority numbers (RPNs).
- **Fault Tree Analysis (FTA):** Uses logical pathways to identify cause-effect relationships leading to system failure.

Auditors must ensure RCA outcomes are evidence-based, documented, and validated for effectiveness. CAPA closures should demonstrate that corrective measures directly address the identified root cause and that preventive measures reduce recurrence likelihood.

RCA represents the intersection of analytical rigor and problem-solving discipline. When applied consistently, it enhances system reliability, supports regulatory compliance, and cultivates a culture of continuous improvement across all operational levels.

Quality Tools Integration and Continuous Improvement

Integration of quality tools ensures that auditing outcomes are translated into measurable organizational improvement. Tools such as cause-and-effect diagrams, control charts, Pareto analysis, and scatter plots are most effective when used in combination to identify, analyze, and resolve systemic issues.

Within medical device organizations, integrated quality analysis links data from CAPA, complaints, and audit findings to broader management review and risk management systems. This cross-functional approach aligns with **ISO 13485 Clause 8.5.1**, which requires ongoing improvement of the effectiveness of the QMS through use of quality policy, objectives, audit results, data analysis, and corrective action.

Auditors must understand how these tools interact to support decision-making. For instance:

- SPC trends can trigger root cause analysis.
- Pareto data can prioritize CAPA focus areas.

- FMEA outputs can inform supplier audits or process validations.

The ultimate goal of tool integration is to establish a feedback-driven culture of continual improvement. In such environments, quality metrics are used not only for compliance reporting but also as active drivers of performance optimization, innovation, and long-term regulatory confidence.

Success on the CMDA examination requires both conceptual mastery and analytical application of the Body of Knowledge. The following structured approach supports efficient and comprehensive preparation:

1. **Understand the Framework:** Review all five Chapters—Auditing Fundamentals, Audit and Inspection Processes, QMS Requirements, Technical Device Knowledge, and Quality Tools—in sequence.

2. **Focus on Relationships:** Recognize how ISO 13485 clauses correspond to 21 CFR 820 subparts and how risk management (ISO 14971) integrates into design and production.

3. **Apply Knowledge Practically:** Work through case scenarios simulating real audits, interpreting evidence and classifying findings.

4. **Use Spaced Repetition:** Review summaries and glossary terms multiple times per week to enhance retention.

5. **Practice Time Management:** Simulate exam conditions—145 multiple-choice questions in 4.5 hours—allocating approximately two minutes per question.

6. **Analyze Sample Questions:** Pay attention to those requiring judgment rather than recall; these test the application of auditing principles.

Finally, maintain composure during the examination. Analytical reasoning and attention to evidence often outweigh rote memorization. Candidates who can synthesize concepts across Chapters are best positioned for success.

Chapter 6 – Practice Questions

Questions (1-100)

Q1. Which of the following best defines a first-party audit?

A. An audit performed by a regulatory body
B. An internal audit conducted by the organization itself
C. A supplier audit performed by a customer
D. An audit for product certification

Q2. Which principle of auditing ensures auditors act independently and without bias?

A. Due professional care
B. Integrity
C. Fair presentation
D. Confidentiality

Q3. Which audit type focuses primarily on verifying a supplier's ability to meet contractual or regulatory requirements?

A. System audit
B. Second-party audit
C. Process audit
D. Product audit

Q4. Which document typically outlines audit scope, objectives, criteria, and team members before audit execution?

A. Audit summary report
B. Audit checklist
C. Audit plan
D. Corrective action plan

Q5. What is the primary purpose of an audit checklist?

A. To record nonconformities
B. To guide consistent evidence collection
C. To summarize audit findings
D. To set audit objectives

Q6. Which term describes the auditor's professional obligation to apply diligence, skill, and judgment?

A. Confidentiality
B. Fair presentation
C. Due professional care
D. Objectivity

Q7. Which of the following is not a typical output of the audit opening meeting?

A. Confirmation of audit scope
B. Agreement on audit schedule
C. Presentation of preliminary findings
D. Introduction of audit team members

Q8. What should auditors do when potential evidence conflicts between different sources?

A. Ignore the inconsistency
B. Record the disagreement but conclude immediately
C. Investigate further until evidence is corroborated
D. Ask management to decide the conclusion

Q9. Confidential information obtained during an audit must be handled according to which key principle?

A. Transparency
B. Integrity
C. Confidentiality
D. Fair presentation

Q10. Which type of audit evidence is most reliable for confirming compliance?
A. Verbal statements from staff
B. Observation of activities
C. Documentation and records
D. Auditor assumptions

Q11. What is the main role of the lead auditor during an audit?
A. To perform data entry
B. To authorize the certification decision
C. To coordinate audit activities and ensure objectives are met
D. To approve corrective actions

Q12. What distinguishes an audit finding from an observation?
A. Findings are informal notes; observations are major nonconformities
B. Findings are conclusions based on evidence; observations are improvement suggestions
C. Findings are always positive; observations are negative
D. There is no difference

Q13. Why must auditors avoid auditing their own work areas?
A. To reduce workload
B. To maintain independence and objectivity
C. To comply with labor laws
D. To minimize training requirements

Q14. Which of the following best defines audit criteria?
A. Procedures used during audit performance
B. Evidence collected from interviews
C. Standards or requirements against which evidence is compared
D. Auditor's personal opinion

Q15. Which activity typically occurs during the audit closing meeting?
A. Development of audit plan
B. Discussion of preliminary findings and next steps
C. Review of audit schedule
D. Selection of audit team members

Q16. Which document usually authorizes the audit to proceed within an organization?
A. Audit checklist
B. Audit charter or schedule approval
C. Audit questionnaire
D. Audit closing report

Q17. Which competency is essential for an auditor to interpret evidence effectively?
A. Familiarity with accounting
B. Technical and process knowledge
C. Marketing experience
D. Personal relationships with staff

Q18. Which phrase best describes fair presentation in auditing?
A. Highlighting only major findings
B. Avoiding documentation of negative results
C. Using management's preferred format

D. Reporting results truthfully and completely without bias

Q19. When an auditor identifies a nonconformance, what should be the immediate next step?

A. Assign corrective action responsibility
B. Document the finding with supporting evidence
C. Debate the issue with management
D. Halt the audit process

Q20. Which attribute is most critical for maintaining auditor credibility?

A. Assertiveness
B. Friendliness
C. Objectivity
D. Seniority

Q21. Which of the following best defines audit scope?

A. The time required to perform the audit
B. The boundaries and extent of audit coverage
C. The qualification of the audit team
D. The results of the previous audit

Q22. Which activity demonstrates objective evidence in an audit?

A. Auditor's assumption about performance
B. Management's verbal assurance
C. Verified calibration record for inspection equipment
D. Auditor's interpretation of staff intent

Q23. The audit criteria for a supplier quality system audit would most likely include:

A. Internal financial data
B. ISO 13485 and contract terms
C. Marketing literature
D. Employee satisfaction surveys

Q24. Which of the following represents a preventive purpose of auditing?

A. Identifying nonconformances after product release
B. Verifying supplier invoices
C. Detecting potential weaknesses before failure occurs
D. Measuring financial performance

Q25. What is the most appropriate auditor action when discovering a serious safety violation during an audit?

A. Ignore it until the closing meeting
B. Stop the audit and immediately report it to management
C. Document it quietly for later review
D. Discuss it informally with the auditee

Q26. Which of the following statements about audit sampling is most accurate?

A. It should only be used in large audits
B. It replaces the need for objective evidence
C. It allows auditors to draw conclusions from representative data
D. It guarantees 100% accuracy

Q27. Which party is primarily responsible for implementing corrective actions after an audit?

A. The auditor
B. The audit sponsor
C. The auditee organization
D. The certification body

Q28. What should an auditor do when encountering hostility or resistance from an auditee?

A. End the audit immediately
B. Report the behavior without discussion
C. Maintain professionalism, de-escalate, and continue fact-finding objectively
D. Respond defensively

Q29. Which statement best reflects the auditor's obligation regarding due care?
A. Auditors are only responsible for major nonconformities
B. Auditors must act diligently, using sound judgment and professional competence
C. Due care applies only to financial audits
D. Due care is optional in internal audits

Q30. In auditing, "risk-based thinking" primarily helps auditors to:
A. Avoid planning activities
B. Prioritize audit focus on areas of greatest potential impact
C. Simplify report writing
D. Increase the number of samples collected

Q31. Which situation would be classified as a major nonconformance?
A. Minor documentation omission
B. Single late training record
C. Systemic failure to validate manufacturing processes
D. Typographical error in a report

Q32. Which of the following describes an auditor bias?
A. Following evidence objectively
B. Forming conclusions before gathering complete evidence
C. Documenting all findings fairly
D. Using multiple data sources for verification

Q33. The audit trail primarily serves to:
A. Track corrective action progress
B. Document evidence supporting audit findings
C. Record team attendance
D. List audit expenses

Q34. What distinguishes a desk audit from an on-site audit?
A. Desk audits review documentation remotely
B. Desk audits involve physical inspections
C. Desk audits require travel
D. Desk audits exclude data review

Q35. Which key competency enables auditors to formulate clear, concise audit reports?
A. Technical writing and analytical ability
B. Product design experience
C. Marketing communication skills
D. Sales negotiation techniques

Q36. The audit program manager is responsible for:
A. Conducting all audits personally
B. Managing schedules, resources, and overall audit performance
C. Reviewing supplier invoices
D. Approving design changes

Q37. Which characteristic most strengthens auditor credibility during interviews?
A. Assertive questioning
B. Active listening and professional respect
C. Rapid conclusions

D. Avoiding eye contact

Q38. The term traceability in auditing refers to:

A. Tracking nonconformances through supply chain logistics

B. The ability to link evidence directly to audit criteria and findings

C. Managing records of past certifications

D. Ensuring anonymity of data sources

Q39. What is the primary advantage of team auditing versus individual auditing?

A. It shortens total audit time

B. It reduces communication requirements

C. It combines diverse expertise and perspectives

D. It eliminates reporting needs

Q40. What should the auditor do if a finding's significance is uncertain during an audit?

A. Omit it from the report

B. Discuss it with the lead auditor or team for consensus

C. Classify it immediately as minor

D. Ask the auditee for classification

Q41. Which of the following is not an example of a second-party audit?

A. A manufacturer auditing its supplier's QMS

B. A customer evaluating a subcontractor's compliance

C. A regulator inspecting a notified body

D. A distributor assessing a vendor's process control

Q42. During an internal audit, the auditor notices incomplete device history records but no evidence of released defective product. What is the most appropriate classification of this issue?

A. Major nonconformance

B. Minor nonconformance

C. Observation

D. Opportunity for improvement

Q43. A lead auditor is planning an audit of a sterilization process that involves multiple subcontractors. Which planning step is most critical?

A. Reviewing calibration logs

B. Clarifying scope boundaries for each subcontractor

C. Interviewing operators in advance

D. Performing the audit unannounced

Q44. You are leading an internal audit and observe that the calibration stickers on several instruments have expired. The production supervisor claims recalibration was done but not recorded. What should you do next?

A. Accept the verbal explanation

B. Verify calibration certificates and records

C. Issue a major nonconformance immediately

D. Stop the audit

Q45. An auditor finds two minor documentation errors in a controlled procedure during a routine audit. The process otherwise meets requirements. What is the best response?

A. Report it as major nonconformance

B. Record an observation for process improvement

C. Ignore it

D. Escalate to management immediately

Q46. Which of the following demonstrates compliance with ISO 19011's principle of independence?

A. Having the quality manager audit their own department

B. Selecting auditors based on convenience
C. Allowing auditors to adjust criteria during the audit
D. Assigning auditors external to the process being audited

Q47. During an audit of complaint handling, the auditor observes missing investigation reports for several complaints. Management states that informal verbal investigations were conducted. What should the auditor conclude?

A. Accept verbal assurance since no harm occurred
B. Raise a major nonconformance for inadequate documentation
C. Recommend verbal approvals
D. Note an opportunity for improvement

Q48. Why is communication skill critical during the audit process?

A. It ensures faster report approval
B. It promotes open, factual discussion and minimizes defensiveness
C. It replaces technical expertise
D. It is optional when using checklists

Q49. What is the main purpose of an audit follow-up?

A. To reopen closed nonconformances
B. To verify the effectiveness of corrective actions taken
C. To train new auditors
D. To reschedule future audits

Q50. A supplier claims to comply with ISO 13485 but refuses to share records due to confidentiality. How should the auditor respond?

A. Accept the claim and move on
B. Terminate the audit immediately
C. Explain that evidence is required and discuss acceptable alternatives, such as redacted records
D. Report the supplier for noncompliance

Q51. Which of the following best defines objectivity in auditing?

A. Avoiding documentation of nonconformities
B. Forming conclusions solely based on verifiable evidence
C. Relying on management input
D. Adjusting findings to match expectations

Q52. During an audit interview, a line operator provides information that contradicts a written SOP. What should the auditor do?

A. Dismiss the operator's statement
B. Report it as nonconformance immediately
C. Compare statements with records and observe actual practices
D. Ask the supervisor to discipline the operator

Q53. What is the main purpose of conducting opening meetings during audits?

A. To finalize audit findings
B. To establish rapport, confirm logistics, and explain objectives
C. To train the auditee staff
D. To issue corrective actions

Q54. You are auditing document control and notice an outdated procedure still being used in one department. The auditee insists the update was distributed last week. What should you request?

A. A copy of the current document distribution record
B. A verbal assurance from the auditee
C. Management approval to ignore it
D. Evidence from another department

Q55. What is the key distinction between audit objectives and audit criteria?
A. Objectives describe what to achieve; criteria define what to compare against
B. Objectives and criteria are identical
C. Objectives are standards; criteria are methods
D. Objectives apply only to suppliers
Q56. While auditing a documentation system, an auditor finds that SOPs lack approval signatures but contain correct revision dates. What should be concluded?
A. Documentation process partially meets requirements
B. No issue exists
C. Audit should stop
D. Process fully compliant
Q57. Which of the following best describes an audit program?
A. A set of audit checklists
B. The overall system for planning and managing multiple audits
C. A single audit report
D. A list of corrective actions
Q58. A junior auditor on your team disagrees with your classification of a finding as "major." How should this be handled?
A. Dismiss the disagreement
B. Seek consensus through discussion and criteria review
C. Report the auditor to management
D. Change classification to avoid conflict
Q59. What is the main purpose of the audit closing meeting?
A. To negotiate corrective actions
B. To present findings and clarify next steps
C. To collect audit fees
D. To revise the audit plan
Q60. During a surveillance audit, you find multiple expired training records for operators. Management argues they are "experienced enough." What should you conclude?
A. Accept the justification
B. Ignore since no defects were found
C. Offer training advice
D. Record a nonconformance for noncompliance with training procedure
Q61. An audit team is reviewing CAPA effectiveness from a previous finding. Records show corrective actions were implemented but not verified. What conclusion is most appropriate?
A. CAPA closed successfully
B. CAPA incomplete—verification missing
C. CAPA unnecessary
D. CAPA effective by assumption
Q62. What is the auditor's primary responsibility regarding risk communication during the audit?
A. Quantify risk levels numerically
B. Escalate high-risk findings promptly to management
C. Perform risk mitigation activities
D. Ignore risk until final reporting
Q63. During an audit of document control, the auditor finds employees using uncontrolled copies of SOPs. What should be the next step?
A. Confiscate the documents
B. Ask employees to discard them

C. Document a nonconformance for use of uncontrolled documents
D. Ignore since procedures are accurate

Q64. What defines audit effectiveness?
A. The number of nonconformances identified
B. Completion within schedule
C. Achievement of planned objectives and contribution to improvement
D. Minimal communication with auditees

Q65. A new auditor is unsure how to handle incomplete responses during interviews. What guidance should the lead auditor provide?
A. Accept partial answers
B. Probe respectfully with open-ended questions
C. Skip the topic
D. Demand written statements

Q66. Which of the following most improves audit consistency between different auditors?
A. Allowing each auditor to define methods
B. Standardized checklists and clear criteria
C. Independent personal judgment
D. Fewer audits per year

Q67. During an audit of training records, the auditor finds that signatures are missing but electronic approvals are recorded. What should be concluded?
A. Process compliant if e-signature system validated
B. Records invalid without ink signature
C. Nonconformance always required
D. No verification needed

Q68. Which audit principle promotes truthful, accurate reporting of findings?
A. Confidentiality
B. Fair presentation
C. Independence
D. Due care

Q69. An auditee insists that a repeated documentation issue "is only cosmetic." However, similar errors appeared in past audits. What classification is most appropriate?
A. Minor
B. Observation
C. Major—systemic recurrence
D. Opportunity for improvement

Q70. What is the most significant risk when auditors fail to maintain independence?
A. Longer audits
B. Reduced cost savings
C. Loss of credibility and invalid audit results
D. Increased report detail

Q71. You are assigned to audit a department you previously supervised. What should you do?
A. Proceed since you understand the process well
B. Request reassignment to maintain independence
C. Audit only the parts you managed
D. Ignore potential bias

Q72. Which quality principle most aligns with the auditor's obligation to act ethically and avoid conflicts of interest?
A. Leadership

B. Integrity
C. Continual improvement
D. Evidence-based decision-making

Q73. An auditor observes incomplete training for personnel conducting process validation. Management claims they "learned on the job." How should the auditor classify this?

A. Major nonconformance—training not documented or verified
B. Minor nonconformance
C. Observation only
D. Not applicable

Q74. Which of the following elements is essential in an audit report?

A. Personal opinions
B. Detailed cost analysis
C. Objective findings linked to criteria
D. Employee names in full

Q75. While reviewing supplier evaluation files, the auditor finds no documentation of risk assessment for new suppliers. What should the auditor do?

A. Record a nonconformance for missing risk-based evaluation
B. Assume approval was verbal
C. Accept long-term supplier history
D. Recommend postponement of audit

Q76. Why are audit field notes important?

A. They replace the final report
B. They serve as confidential drafts for management
C. They provide supporting detail and traceability for audit findings
D. They are optional in ISO audits

Q77. During a team audit, two auditors disagree on whether evidence demonstrates a nonconformance. How should the lead auditor resolve this?

A. Choose the more experienced auditor's view
B. Seek consensus using evidence and criteria
C. Vote by majority
D. Postpone decision indefinitely

Q78. What is the main goal of the audit opening statement delivered by the lead auditor?

A. To present audit findings
B. To outline audit objectives, criteria, and logistics clearly
C. To justify auditor expenses
D. To summarize last year's performance

Q79. An auditor discovers that an internal audit program has not been updated in three years despite process changes. What should be concluded?

A. No issue if audits are still performed
B. Nonconformance—program not maintained to reflect current operations
C. Acceptable with justification
D. Observation only

Q80. Which of the following actions most enhances audit credibility during regulatory inspection readiness audits?

A. Ignoring minor issues
B. Relying on management input
C. Using personal judgment
D. Basing conclusions on documented, verifiable evidence

Q81. Which step should be completed first when developing an audit plan?
A. Assign team roles
B. Identify audit objectives and scope
C. Schedule closing meeting
D. Draft checklist questions
Q82. A lead auditor receives notice that a critical process owner will be on leave during the scheduled audit. What should be done?
A. Cancel the audit
B. Proceed without interviewing substitutes
C. Adjust the plan to include alternate qualified personnel
D. Ignore the absence
Q83. The opening meeting primarily serves to:
A. Present audit results
B. Verify logistics, scope, and roles with the auditee
C. Discuss CAPA history
D. Deliver auditor training
Q84. During a supplier audit, you discover production occurring outside the documented cleanroom area. What is the best immediate action?
A. Ignore since cleanliness seems adequate
B. Halt all operations
C. Document objective evidence and inform management during audit
D. Discuss privately after report issuance
Q85. Which document best defines audit criteria?
A. Internal checklist only
B. Applicable standards, regulations, or procedures
C. Auditor's personal experience
D. Previous audit reports
Q86. Mid-audit, a team member identifies a potential nonconformance but lacks sufficient proof. What should the lead auditor instruct?
A. Conclude it as confirmed
B. Gather more evidence before classifying
C. Delete the note
D. Escalate immediately as major
Q87. Which activity occurs during audit performance?
A. Scheduling closing meeting
B. Reviewing and verifying objective evidence
C. Final report distribution
D. Corrective-action approval
Q88. An auditee challenges an auditor's finding during the closing meeting. What is the proper auditor response?
A. Argue firmly until accepted
B. Remove the finding
C. Explain evidence and criteria calmly, inviting additional documented proof
D. End discussion immediately
Q89. What distinguishes process audits from system audits?
A. Process audits focus on a single activity flow; system audits evaluate the entire QMS structure
B. Process audits are external only
C. System audits require fewer records

D. No distinction exists

Q90. You find evidence suggesting potential data integrity tampering in batch records. What should be done first?

A. Confront the operator
B. Suspend the audit
C. Notify the lead auditor and document evidence securely
D. Ignore until next audit

Q91. Which section of an audit report is most useful for management review?

A. List of auditee names
B. Executive summary with findings and recommendations
C. Detailed checklist answers only
D. Auditor travel notes

Q92. An audit team observes corrective actions implemented but recurring minor issues in the same area. What should they conclude?

A. CAPA fully effective
B. CAPA not verified for long-term sustainability
C. CAPA unnecessary
D. Evidence invalid

Q93. In planning audits under an annual program, which factor should drive priority?

A. Auditor availability
B. Risk level and regulatory impact of processes
C. Rotational fairness
D. Alphabetical department listing

Q94. While auditing supplier controls, the auditor discovers that approved vendor lists are outdated by a year. What should be reported?

A. Observation only
B. Major supplier violation automatically
C. Acceptable due to historical stability
D. Nonconformance—failure to maintain current approved supplier list

Q95. What is the primary purpose of a closing meeting?

A. Negotiate penalties
B. Present findings, obtain acknowledgment, and clarify next steps
C. Collect evidence
D. Train auditees

Q96. During a regulatory inspection simulation, the auditor notices operators using outdated batch records. What should be the immediate auditor action?

A. Note it quietly
B. Stop production instantly without authority
C. Record objective evidence and escalate through audit lead
D. Ignore if quality unaffected

Q97. Which of the following enhances reliability of audit conclusions?

A. Evidence from one interview only
B. Triangulation—using multiple sources of corroborating data
C. Auditor intuition
D. Excluding conflicting data

Q98. A lead auditor completes a multi-site audit and identifies systemic issues across all locations. What reporting approach is best?

A. Issue separate reports per site without linkage

B. Consolidate common findings under a corporate summary report
C. Report only the largest site
D. Ignore smaller sites' data

Q99. Which element must be included in every audit checklist?
A. Company vision statement
B. Audit questions linked to criteria references
C. Employee personal notes
D. Budget estimates

Q100. A follow-up audit reveals that a corrective action was closed administratively but not implemented. What should the auditor record?
A. No finding—closure documented
B. Major nonconformance—ineffective CAPA implementation
C. Observation only
D. Opportunity for improvement

Answer key and Explanation (1-100)

Q1. Answer: B
Explanation: A first-party audit is an internal self-assessment conducted by the organization to verify its conformance to requirements and readiness for external evaluation. It measures internal compliance, supports continual improvement, and prepares for second- or third-party audits.
SubChapter: Audit Types and Purpose

Q2. Answer: B
Explanation: Integrity requires auditors to conduct activities honestly, objectively, and without conflicts of interest, forming the foundation for trust in audit conclusions and impartial results. Independence in mindset and action supports the credibility of the entire audit process.
SubChapter: Auditing Principles

Q3. Answer: B
Explanation: A second-party audit is performed by a customer on its supplier to evaluate compliance with purchase agreements, quality expectations, and regulatory criteria, ensuring reliable sourcing and supplier performance aligned with organizational quality goals.
SubChapter: Audit Classification

Q4. Answer: C
Explanation: The audit plan provides a structured roadmap for audit activities, defining what will be assessed, by whom, and when. It ensures adequate preparation, time allocation, and transparency among the audit team and auditee to achieve efficient, effective execution.
SubChapter: Audit Planning

Q5. Answer: B
Explanation: An audit checklist serves as a structured guide to verify conformance with criteria, helping auditors systematically collect evidence, stay aligned with scope, and maintain objectivity throughout audit performance and documentation.
SubChapter: Audit Tools

Q6. Answer: C
Explanation: Due professional care means auditors must exercise competence, caution, and thoroughness during all audit activities. This includes accurate evidence evaluation, objective judgment, and ethical decision-making in compliance with professional standards and organizational policies.
SubChapter: Auditor Conduct

Q7. Answer: C
Explanation: Preliminary findings are discussed later during the closing meeting, not at opening. The opening session clarifies scope, logistics, team introductions, and communication protocols to ensure alignment between auditors and auditees before audit activities begin.
SubChapter: Audit Execution

Q8. Answer: C
Explanation: Auditors must validate conflicting evidence through additional investigation or sampling to ensure conclusions are accurate, objective, and based on reliable, corroborated data, safeguarding the credibility of audit findings and reports.
SubChapter: Evidence Evaluation

Q9. Answer: C
Explanation: The confidentiality principle ensures auditors protect sensitive information acquired during the audit and refrain from disclosing it without authorization. This ethical requirement preserves trust, organizational reputation, and legal compliance across regulated industries.
SubChapter: Professional Ethics

Q10. Answer: C

Explanation: Documentary evidence such as records, logs, and approved procedures provide verifiable, traceable proof of compliance, carrying higher reliability than verbal statements or assumptions. Observations complement but rarely replace formal documented evidence.
SubChapter: Audit Evidence

Q11. Answer: C

Explanation: The lead auditor plans, directs, and manages audit execution, ensuring all team members follow the plan, evidence is properly reviewed, and findings align with audit scope and objectives. Leadership ensures consistency and procedural control.
SubChapter: Audit Roles and Responsibilities

Q12. Answer: B

Explanation: An audit finding is a formal conclusion referencing conformance or nonconformance with criteria, while an observation highlights potential improvement areas or minor risks. Differentiating them supports balanced reporting and continuous improvement.
SubChapter: Audit Reporting

Q13. Answer: B

Explanation: Independence is essential to prevent bias or conflicts of interest. Auditors cannot evaluate processes they manage, as doing so compromises objectivity, undermining credibility of audit conclusions and stakeholder confidence.
SubChapter: Auditor Independence

Q14. Answer: C

Explanation: Audit criteria represent the reference standards, policies, or regulations used to assess compliance. They provide the baseline for evaluating objective evidence and determining conformance or nonconformance in a structured, defensible manner.
SubChapter: Audit Criteria and Scope

Q15. Answer: B

Explanation: The closing meeting summarizes findings, clarifies nonconformities, and outlines next actions for corrective measures or follow-up. It provides transparency, ensures understanding by the auditee, and finalizes communication of audit outcomes.
SubChapter: Audit Reporting and Closure

Q16. Answer: B

Explanation: An approved audit charter or schedule formally authorizes audit execution, identifying responsible parties, timing, and scope. It signals management commitment and ensures auditees are aware of and prepared for the audit activity.
SubChapter: Audit Authorization

Q17. Answer: B

Explanation: Auditors must understand relevant processes, standards, and technologies to interpret evidence accurately. Technical competence allows them to evaluate compliance with system requirements, identify risks, and make valid, defensible audit conclusions.
SubChapter: Auditor Competence

Q18. Answer: D

Explanation: Fair presentation demands auditors report audit findings accurately, objectively, and completely, including both positive and negative results, to ensure credibility and transparency in audit reports and stakeholder communications.
SubChapter: Audit Ethics and Integrity

Q19. Answer: B

Explanation: The auditor should document the nonconformance clearly, referencing specific evidence and criteria violated. Accurate documentation ensures traceability, facilitates corrective action, and maintains professional integrity in audit records.

SubChapter: Audit Documentation

Q20. Answer: C

Explanation: Objectivity ensures auditors remain impartial, evaluating evidence based solely on facts and established criteria. It underpins audit integrity, accuracy, and acceptance of conclusions by management and regulatory authorities alike.

SubChapter: Auditor Attributes

Q21. Answer: B

Explanation: Audit scope defines what the audit will cover—specific processes, departments, and timeframes—ensuring focus and preventing unnecessary expansion. Clear scope boundaries help manage expectations and maintain relevance to the audit objectives and criteria.

SubChapter: Audit Scope Definition

Q22. Answer: C

Explanation: Objective evidence is verifiable information based on records, statements of fact, or observations that can be confirmed independently. Calibration certificates, training records, and inspection logs are examples of such tangible evidence supporting audit findings.

SubChapter: Audit Evidence Collection

Q23. Answer: B

Explanation: Supplier audits assess compliance with applicable standards such as ISO 13485 and contractual obligations. These criteria guide evidence collection and ensure the supplier's quality system meets regulatory and customer expectations.

SubChapter: Audit Criteria and Standards

Q24. Answer: C

Explanation: Preventive auditing proactively identifies areas of risk or process weakness before defects or regulatory violations occur. This enhances continuous improvement, compliance, and operational reliability by encouraging early corrective actions.

SubChapter: Audit Purpose and Value

Q25. Answer: B

Explanation: Serious safety violations must be escalated immediately to responsible management to prevent harm or regulatory exposure. Auditors prioritize safety and compliance above procedural convenience or audit schedule adherence.

SubChapter: Ethics and Professional Conduct

Q26. Answer: C

Explanation: Sampling enables efficient auditing by evaluating representative data subsets rather than exhaustive reviews. When properly selected, samples yield reliable conclusions without excessive resource use, balancing audit thoroughness with practicality.

SubChapter: Sampling and Evidence Evaluation

Q27. Answer: C

Explanation: The auditee is responsible for developing and implementing corrective actions to address nonconformities. The auditor's role is to verify completion and effectiveness but not to prescribe or execute corrective measures.

SubChapter: Corrective Action Responsibility

Q28. Answer: C

Explanation: Auditors must remain calm, impartial, and focused on evidence. Professional communication and de-escalation protect the audit's integrity and credibility while ensuring respect and cooperation between auditor and auditee.

SubChapter: Auditor Behavior and Communication

Q29. Answer: B

Explanation: Due professional care requires auditors to act competently, verify evidence carefully, and exercise balanced judgment. It is a universal principle across audit types, ensuring accuracy and ethical consistency in findings and conclusions.
SubChapter: Auditor Professionalism

Q30. Answer: B

Explanation: Risk-based thinking allows auditors to allocate time and resources toward areas that pose the highest compliance or safety risks. This strategic approach enhances audit effectiveness and aligns with modern ISO 9001 and 13485 methodologies.
SubChapter: Audit Risk Awareness

Q31. Answer: C

Explanation: Major nonconformances indicate systemic or serious process breakdowns affecting compliance or product quality. They require prompt corrective action and management attention due to their significant potential impact on safety or regulatory status.
SubChapter: Audit Findings Classification

Q32. Answer: B

Explanation: Auditor bias occurs when conclusions are influenced by preconceived opinions or incomplete evidence. Avoiding bias ensures objectivity and credibility of audit results, preserving the integrity of the entire audit process.
SubChapter: Auditor Ethics

Q33. Answer: B

Explanation: The audit trail provides traceable documentation linking findings to supporting evidence. It enables verification, transparency, and defensibility of audit results during internal reviews or external regulatory evaluations.
SubChapter: Audit Documentation and Traceability

Q34. Answer: A

Explanation: A desk audit examines records and documentation without visiting the site, often used for supplier pre-assessments or follow-up reviews. On-site audits involve field verification through interviews and process observation.
SubChapter: Audit Methods

Q35. Answer: A

Explanation: Effective report writing requires clarity, objectivity, and analytical organization. Auditors must present evidence-based conclusions using precise, neutral language that communicates results effectively to both technical and managerial audiences.
SubChapter: Audit Reporting Skills

Q36. Answer: B

Explanation: The audit program manager oversees the organizational audit framework, ensuring audits are planned, resourced, and executed per objectives and timelines. This role also monitors auditor competence and continual improvement within the audit program.
SubChapter: Audit Program Management

Q37. Answer: B

Explanation: Effective auditors use active listening to build rapport and obtain complete, accurate responses. Respectful, patient communication enhances cooperation, reduces defensiveness, and increases the reliability of collected evidence.
SubChapter: Interview Techniques

Q38. Answer: B

Explanation: Traceability ensures all findings are linked back to their evidence and associated audit criteria, providing a clear verification path for reviewers or regulators to confirm audit accuracy and completeness.

SubChapter: Evidence Management

Q39. Answer: C

Explanation: Team audits leverage multiple competencies and viewpoints, improving depth and accuracy of evaluations, especially in complex or multidisciplinary systems. Collaboration enhances coverage and minimizes oversight risk.

SubChapter: Audit Team Dynamics

Q40. Answer: B

Explanation: Ambiguous findings should be reviewed collaboratively to ensure accurate classification and consistency with audit criteria. Consensus decision-making maintains fairness and prevents overstatement or understatement of compliance issues.

SubChapter: Team Collaboration and Decision-Making

Q41. Answer: C

Explanation: A regulator inspection is a third-party audit, not a second-party. Second-party audits are conducted by customers or organizations on suppliers to ensure quality and contractual compliance within supply chains.

SubChapter: Audit Relationships and Types

Q42. Answer: B

Explanation: Incomplete documentation that does not directly impact product quality is typically a minor nonconformance. It still violates procedural requirements but indicates a localized or administrative lapse, not a systemic control failure.

SubChapter: Finding Classification and Risk Assessment

Q43. Answer: B

Explanation: When multiple parties are involved, defining clear scope boundaries and responsibilities ensures each subcontractor's processes are properly evaluated and avoids overlap or omission of key activities.

SubChapter: Audit Planning and Scope Control

Q44. Answer: B

Explanation: Verification of records is necessary before classification. Auditor conclusions must rely on documented, objective evidence, not verbal claims. If records are absent, the issue may escalate to a formal nonconformance.

SubChapter: Evidence Verification and Objectivity

Q45. Answer: B

Explanation: Minor inconsistencies that do not compromise compliance should be recorded as observations, encouraging corrective or preventive action without formal nonconformance status. This promotes continuous improvement culture.

SubChapter: Audit Reporting Judgment

Q46. Answer: D

Explanation: Independence ensures auditors are free from bias or direct responsibility for the audited activities. Selecting auditors external to the process maintains objectivity and enhances credibility of results.

SubChapter: Audit Ethics and Independence

Q47. Answer: B

Explanation: Complaint investigations must be documented under 21 CFR 820.198. Absence of records violates regulatory requirements, constituting a major nonconformance affecting compliance credibility and traceability.

SubChapter: Documentation and Regulatory Compliance

Q48. Answer: B

Explanation: Effective communication allows auditors to extract accurate information, clarify misunderstandings, and foster cooperation. Constructive dialogue reduces resistance and ensures findings are understood and accepted by auditees.
SubChapter: Auditor Interpersonal Competence
Q49. Answer: B
Explanation: Follow-up ensures corrective actions are implemented and effective in preventing recurrence. It validates that the organization has resolved the root cause and achieved sustainable improvement.
SubChapter: Post-Audit Verification
Q50. Answer: C
Explanation: Auditors must balance confidentiality and evidence requirements. Negotiating alternate verification methods, like redacted documents or on-screen reviews, maintains transparency and protects sensitive data while completing the audit.
SubChapter: Confidentiality and Evidence Handling
Q51. Answer: B
Explanation: Objectivity ensures audit conclusions stem strictly from evidence, not personal preference or external influence. It upholds impartiality and reinforces the reliability of the entire audit process.
SubChapter: Auditing Principles
Q52. Answer: C
Explanation: Discrepancies between documentation and practice must be verified through observation and record review. The auditor's role is to confirm evidence objectively before drawing conclusions.
SubChapter: Evidence Corroboration
Q53. Answer: B
Explanation: Opening meetings ensure all parties understand audit purpose, scope, schedule, and communication channels, promoting transparency and cooperation from the start of the audit.
SubChapter: Audit Execution Procedures
Q54. Answer: A
Explanation: Verifying document distribution ensures controlled processes are effectively implemented. The auditor must confirm that updates are formally issued and acknowledged organization-wide to prevent compliance lapses.
SubChapter: Document Control Verification
Q55. Answer: A
Explanation: Objectives outline the audit's intended outcomes—such as compliance assessment or improvement—while criteria are the standards or regulations used for comparison. Both are critical to audit planning and evaluation.
SubChapter: Audit Framework
Q56. Answer: A
Explanation: Missing approvals indicate incomplete document control, even if revision tracking exists. This suggests procedural gaps requiring corrective action to ensure compliance with ISO 13485 documentation controls.
SubChapter: Document Management and Conformance
Q57. Answer: B
Explanation: An audit program is a structured framework encompassing planning, scheduling, resourcing, and evaluating multiple audits to ensure systematic, consistent compliance monitoring across the organization.
SubChapter: Audit Program Structure
Q58. Answer: B

Explanation: Team alignment on classification ensures consistency and defensibility. Discussion based on evidence and objective criteria reinforces collaborative learning and accurate reporting.
SubChapter: Team Collaboration and Consensus
Q59. Answer: B
Explanation: The closing meeting summarizes findings, clarifies nonconformities, and establishes timelines for corrective actions, ensuring shared understanding between auditor and auditee.
SubChapter: Audit Reporting and Closure
Q60. Answer: D
Explanation: Documented evidence of training compliance is mandatory. Lack of current records violates QMS requirements and regulatory expectations, making this a nonconformance regardless of operator experience.
SubChapter: Competence and Record Control
Q61. Answer: B
Explanation: Verification confirms whether implemented corrective actions resolved the root cause. Absence of verification evidence means the CAPA process is incomplete, potentially allowing recurrence of the issue.
SubChapter: Corrective Action Verification
Q62. Answer: B
Explanation: Auditors must communicate significant or safety-related risks immediately to management to ensure timely action. Transparent risk reporting supports proactive decisions and protects regulatory compliance.
SubChapter: Risk Communication and Ethics
Q63. Answer: C
Explanation: Uncontrolled documents risk the use of outdated information. Auditors must document this as a nonconformance, as it violates ISO 13485 and QMS control requirements for document distribution.
SubChapter: Document Control Compliance
Q64. Answer: C
Explanation: An effective audit fulfills defined objectives, provides actionable insights, and enhances organizational performance or compliance. Success depends on quality, not quantity, of findings.
SubChapter: Audit Performance Evaluation
Q65. Answer: B
Explanation: Open-ended questions encourage detailed, candid responses and reveal deeper process understanding. Skilled interview technique ensures completeness of evidence while maintaining rapport.
SubChapter: Interview Skills and Communication
Q66. Answer: B
Explanation: Standardized checklists and documented criteria ensure uniform interpretation and data collection across auditors, minimizing variability and enhancing repeatability of results.
SubChapter: Audit Standardization and Consistency
Q67. Answer: A
Explanation: Electronic approvals are acceptable when validated per 21 CFR Part 11 and ISO 13485. Validation ensures integrity, authenticity, and traceability of digital records.
SubChapter: Electronic Records and Validation
Q68. Answer: B
Explanation: Fair presentation ensures that findings are reported truthfully and comprehensively, including both positive and negative results, maintaining transparency and professional integrity.
SubChapter: Audit Principles – Fair Presentation
Q69. Answer: C

Explanation: Recurring issues indicate systemic control weakness. A repeated lapse despite prior corrective action elevates the issue's severity to major nonconformance.
SubChapter: Finding Evaluation and Escalation

Q70. Answer: C

Explanation: Independence ensures impartial conclusions. When compromised, audit credibility erodes, findings lose validity, and confidence in results diminishes internally and externally.
SubChapter: Auditor Ethics and Objectivity

Q71. Answer: B

Explanation: Prior responsibility creates a conflict of interest. Requesting reassignment upholds objectivity, preventing bias and ensuring compliance with ISO 19011 independence principles.
SubChapter: Conflict of Interest Management

Q72. Answer: B

Explanation: Integrity drives ethical behavior, transparency, and honesty. It compels auditors to disclose conflicts, maintain confidentiality, and prioritize truthfulness in evidence reporting.
SubChapter: Ethical Conduct

Q73. Answer: A

Explanation: Regulatory frameworks require documented, verified competence for personnel performing validation. Lack of training evidence represents a serious systemic deficiency, qualifying as major nonconformance.
SubChapter: Competence and Qualification Records

Q74. Answer: C

Explanation: Reports must link each finding directly to objective evidence and relevant criteria. This ensures traceability, defensibility, and clear understanding by management.
SubChapter: Audit Reporting Standards

Q75. Answer: A

Explanation: ISO 13485 requires risk-based supplier evaluation. Absence of such documentation violates purchasing control requirements, warranting a nonconformance report.
SubChapter: Supplier Audit and Risk Management

Q76. Answer: C

Explanation: Field notes record real-time evidence, ensuring findings are traceable and verifiable. They strengthen audit defensibility and accuracy during report preparation.
SubChapter: Evidence Documentation

Q77. Answer: B

Explanation: The lead auditor should guide discussion referencing audit criteria and evidence. Consensus-based resolution ensures consistency and balanced judgment within the audit team.
SubChapter: Team Leadership and Consensus Building

Q78. Answer: B

Explanation: The opening statement sets expectations by explaining audit purpose, criteria, scope, methods, and schedule, establishing a cooperative and transparent environment.
SubChapter: Audit Opening Meeting Procedures

Q79. Answer: B

Explanation: Audit programs must be reviewed periodically to remain relevant and risk-based. Failure to update them compromises coverage and violates ISO 19011 guidance.
SubChapter: Audit Program Maintenance

Q80. Answer: D

Explanation: Regulatory and certification bodies rely on objective, verifiable evidence. Conclusions grounded in documented proof uphold audit credibility, reliability, and regulatory defensibility.
SubChapter: Evidence-Based Decision Making

Q81. Answer: B
Explanation: Establishing clear audit objectives and scope defines what will be evaluated, why, and to what extent. This foundation ensures every subsequent planning action—including scheduling, resources, and criteria—aligns with intended outcomes and regulatory expectations.
SubChapter: Audit Planning Sequence
Q82. Answer: C
Explanation: Audits must ensure adequate evidence collection despite personnel changes. Adjusting the plan to include alternate, knowledgeable representatives maintains coverage while preventing schedule disruption or evidence gaps.
SubChapter: Contingency Planning
Q83. Answer: B
Explanation: The opening meeting aligns expectations by confirming audit objectives, scope, criteria, and communication channels. It promotes cooperation, clarifies uncertainties, and sets a transparent tone for efficient audit execution.
SubChapter: Audit Initiation
Q84. Answer: C
Explanation: The auditor must record factual evidence and alert responsible management promptly, as off-controlled-area manufacturing could violate regulatory or QMS controls. Early communication allows corrective containment while maintaining audit objectivity.
SubChapter: On-Site Observation and Escalation
Q85. Answer: B
Explanation: Audit criteria are the authoritative requirements—such as ISO 13485, 21 CFR 820, or corporate SOPs—used to evaluate conformance. They provide the benchmark against which objective evidence is compared to determine compliance status.
SubChapter: Audit Framework Definition
Q86. Answer: B
Explanation: Findings must be evidence-based. The auditor should collect additional documentation, samples, or observations to substantiate or dismiss the concern objectively before formal classification.
SubChapter: Evidence Validation
Q87. Answer: B
Explanation: Audit performance is the execution phase where auditors collect, analyze, and verify objective evidence through interviews, document review, and observation to determine conformity with defined criteria.
SubChapter: Audit Execution
Q88. Answer: C
Explanation: Professional discussion supported by evidence and standards encourages mutual understanding. If valid counter-evidence exists, it can be reviewed objectively before finalizing the report.
SubChapter: Professional Communication and Conflict Resolution
Q89. Answer: A
Explanation: Process audits examine specific operations or sequences for effectiveness and compliance, while system audits assess the overall management system's adequacy and integration.
SubChapter: Audit Type Differentiation
Q90. Answer: C
Explanation: Suspected data falsification requires immediate, confidential escalation to the lead auditor or management. Objective evidence must be preserved without accusation to ensure ethical, compliant handling of possible integrity breaches.
SubChapter: Data Integrity and Ethics

Q91. Answer: B
Explanation: The executive summary concisely presents key findings, trends, and recommendations, enabling management to prioritize resources, evaluate risk, and make informed decisions for corrective or preventive action.
SubChapter: Audit Reporting Structure
Q92. Answer: B
Explanation: Repeated issues indicate insufficient follow-up or ineffective root-cause elimination. The team should note that CAPA verification did not ensure sustained control, signaling the need for deeper cause analysis.
SubChapter: CAPA Effectiveness Evaluation
Q93. Answer: B
Explanation: Risk-based scheduling ensures high-impact or compliance-critical processes receive more frequent audits, aligning with ISO 19011 and FDA risk-management principles for efficient resource allocation.
SubChapter: Risk-Based Audit Planning
Q94. Answer: D
Explanation: Maintaining updated approved-supplier documentation is a QMS requirement. Outdated lists risk purchasing from unqualified vendors, warranting a documented nonconformance for process lapse.
SubChapter: Supplier Evaluation Controls
Q95. Answer: B
Explanation: The closing meeting communicates results, classifications, and action expectations transparently, ensuring mutual understanding and formal acknowledgment by management before final report release.
SubChapter: Audit Closure Protocol
Q96. Answer: C
Explanation: Using obsolete records violates documentation control and could impact product compliance. The auditor must document details factually and notify responsible management via the proper audit chain.
SubChapter: Immediate Escalation Procedures
Q97. Answer: B
Explanation: Triangulation cross-verifies information from documents, observations, and interviews, strengthening conclusion validity and reducing bias in audit interpretation.
SubChapter: Evidence Corroboration
Q98. Answer: B
Explanation: Consolidated reporting highlights systemic weaknesses affecting multiple sites, enabling coordinated corporate corrective action and demonstrating holistic analysis to regulators.
SubChapter: Multi-Site Audit Reporting
Q99. Answer: B
Explanation: Each checklist item should reference applicable clauses or procedures, ensuring traceability between audit questions, criteria, and collected evidence for consistent and objective evaluation.
SubChapter: Checklist Design
Q100. Answer: B
Explanation: Documented closure without action demonstrates systemic weakness in CAPA execution and management oversight, qualifying as a major nonconformance due to failure to verify actual implementation.
SubChapter: Follow-Up Audit Verification

Questions (101-200)

Q101. What is the first section of a complete audit report?

A. Audit summary

B. Audit scope

C. Audit purpose

D. Audit date

Q102. You identify an issue but lack direct evidence. What should be done next?

A. Record assumption

B. Gather data

C. Report finding

D. Skip review

Q103. Which type of audit focuses on verifying compliance to ISO 13485 clauses?

A. Product audit

B. System audit

C. Process audit

D. Desk audit

Q104. The lead auditor is responsible for:

A. Writing SOPs

B. Coordinating team

C. Approving CAPA

D. Issuing penalties

Q105. During a closing meeting, management disputes one major finding. What should the auditor do?

A. Argue firmly

B. Stay silent

C. Discuss evidence

D. Remove finding

Q106. What does MDSAP stand for?

A. Multi-Chapter Safety Audit Program

B. Medical Device Single Audit Program

C. Multi-Department System Audit Process

D. Medical Data System Audit Protocol

Q107. What is the key purpose of audit follow-up?

A. Verify correction

B. Close file

C. Train staff

D. Write SOPs

Q108. A supplier's CAPA plan is delayed by two months. What is the best auditor action?

A. Escalate delay

B. Ignore delay

C. Rewrite CAPA

D. Cancel audit

Q109. Which element should not appear in an audit report?

A. Findings summary

B. Auditor opinions

C. Audit criteria

D. Audit date

Q110. During an MDSAP audit, the team identifies a CAPA that addresses multiple jurisdictions. What should be ensured?
A. Local focus only
B. Jurisdiction coverage
C. One CAPA per site
D. Delay review
Q111. A well-written finding should be:
A. Brief and clear
B. Vague but polite
C. Personal and broad
D. Informal and simple
Q112. You observe operators bypassing data entry steps to save time. What should the auditor do first?
A. Report suspicion
B. Collect evidence
C. Ask management
D. Stop operation
Q113. What is QSIT used for?
A. Training employees
B. Auditing FDA QSR
C. Validating devices
D. Labeling control
Q114. Which step follows audit execution?
A. CAPA follow-up
B. Audit reporting
C. Evidence review
D. Team briefing
Q115. A CAPA was implemented but no verification results exist. What should the auditor conclude?
A. CAPA closed
B. CAPA incomplete
C. CAPA approved
D. CAPA optional
Q116. The most important feature of audit traceability is:
A. Finding linkage
B. Data privacy
C. Cost tracking
D. Auditor listing
Q117. An auditor reports three repeat findings from prior audits. What is the best classification?
A. Minor trend
B. Major system issue
C. Observation only
D. Opportunity area
Q118. What is a nonconformity statement required to include?
A. Who erred
B. Objective evidence
C. Auditor opinion
D. Root cause

Q119. During a follow-up, CAPA records are missing verification results. Management insists verbal confirmation was given. What should be done?
A. Accept verbally
B. Record evidence gap
C. Close CAPA
D. Ignore issue
Q120. Which outcome best defines a successful audit?
A. Many findings
B. Achieved objectives
C. Few reports
D. Fast closure
Q121. Which section confirms audit boundaries?
A. Scope
B. Goals
C. Plan
D. Dates
Q122. A supplier refuses access to maintenance records. What should you do first?
A. Escalate
B. Record
C. Negotiate
D. Ignore
Q123. Which phrase best describes an audit trail?
A. Record path
B. Evidence link
C. Event summary
D. Data map
Q124. A CAPA closure form lists actions complete but no verification field. What should the auditor note?
A. Observation
B. Minor NC
C. Major NC
D. Acceptable
Q125. Which quality ensures audit reports are credible?
A. Accuracy
B. Brevity
C. Tone
D. Layout
Q126. A team auditor records incomplete observation details. What must the lead auditor do?
A. Revise
B. Approve
C. Verify
D. Delete
Q127. Which method confirms CAPA effectiveness?
A. Trend data
B. CAPA form
C. Audit plan
D. SOP check
Q128. During follow-up, audit evidence contradicts CAPA claims. What should be done?

A. Accept
B. Report
C. Discuss
D. Close

Q129. Which attribute defines a good finding statement?

A. Specific
B. Broad
C. Personal
D. Predictive

Q130. You observe operators skip sign-off steps. Evidence photos are taken. What is next?

A. Verify
B. Close
C. Report
D. Store

Q131. What must every audit report include?

A. Date
B. Criteria
C. Title
D. Scope

Q132. A CAPA addresses a labeling issue but fails to analyze root cause. What should the auditor record?

A. Minor NC
B. Major NC
C. Observation
D. Acceptable

Q133. Which metric best shows CAPA trend health?

A. Closure rate
B. Cost spent
C. Staff hours
D. Forms count

Q134. An auditee submits partial records for evidence. What should the auditor request?

A. Remainder
B. Approval
C. Meeting
D. Waiver

Q135. What ensures audit reports remain confidential?

A. Secure storage
B. Broad access
C. Shared emails
D. Cloud posting

Q136. A follow-up audit finds no objective proof of preventive action. What is proper action?

A. Report NC
B. Close CAPA
C. Delay review
D. Accept verbal

Q137. Which tool assists in root-cause analysis?

A. Gantt map
B. Calendar

C. Chart pad
D. Fishbone
Q138. A CAPA remains open for a year without follow-up. What risk exists?
A. Data loss
B. Ineffective system
C. Staff overuse
D. Low audit
Q139. Which principle ensures report statements are fair?
A. Impartiality
B. Integrity
C. Independence
D. Courtesy
Q140. During MDSAP review, you note identical findings repeated in three tasks. What should be concluded?
A. Local issue
B. Systemic trend
C. Minor error
D. Random case
Q141. What defines inspection technique?
A. Observation skill
B. Evaluation method
C. Verification tool
D. Audit checklist
Q142. An auditor must inspect device labeling for accuracy. Which technique is best?
A. Visual check
B. Random test
C. Desk review
D. Verbal query
Q143. What is the main goal of sampling in audits?
A. Save time
B. Represent data
C. Reduce scope
D. Avoid detail
Q144. An auditor selects every 10th batch record to review. Which sampling type is used?
A. Random
B. Systematic
C. Stratified
D. Judgmental
Q145. Which sampling approach best minimizes bias?
A. Random
B. Fixed
C. Rotated
D. Clustered
Q146. During inspection, 2 of 20 samples fail acceptance criteria. What should the auditor do?
A. Expand scope
B. Stop audit
C. Discard data
D. Accept results

Q147. What is the primary purpose of inspection records?
A. Store data
B. Verify trace
C. Document evidence
D. Summarize cost
Q148. An audit of incoming materials reveals no sampling plan in the SOP. What should the auditor note?
A. Major NC
B. Minor NC
C. Observation
D. Acceptable
Q149. What should determine audit sample size?
A. Risk level
B. Staff count
C. Auditor time
D. Record order
Q150. An auditor finds inconsistent calibration logs between shifts. What is the correct action?
A. Verify cause
B. Report issue
C. Ignore logs
D. Delay audit
Q151. What is the main goal of inspection consistency?
A. Uniform results
B. Faster work
C. Higher yield
D. Lower cost
Q152. A reinspection of previously rejected units finds 1 additional defect. What does this imply?
A. Data error
B. Operator skill
C. Normal variance
D. Process drift
Q153. What defines inspection objectivity?
A. Evidence only
B. Personal views
C. Verbal feedback
D. Past reports
Q154. Auditors reviewing supplier inspection data note missing signatures on 5 of 10 records. What should be done?
A. Raise NC
B. Verify proof
C. Note comment
D. Skip file
Q155. What is the role of audit checklists in inspections?
A. Guide focus
B. Record cost
C. Limit time
D. Replace plan
Q156. A process audit uses 100% inspection for every lot. What issue may arise?

A. Resource strain
B. Quality gain
C. Cost drop
D. Speed rise

Q157. Which factor most influences sampling confidence level?

A. Sample size
B. Staff count
C. Report length
D. Cost plan

Q158. A calibration audit shows consistent date errors across all logs. What is the likely issue?

A. Normal delay
B. Operator bias
C. Data theft
D. Template flaw

Q159. What ensures reporting consistency across auditors?

A. Common format
B. Team rotation
C. Data variety
D. Brief reports

Q160. During MDSAP inspection, results vary between auditors using different checklists. What should leadership do?

A. Harmonize tool
B. Replace staff
C. Reduce audits
D. Ignore variance

Q161. What defines a process-based audit?

A. Flow review
B. Record scan
C. Policy check
D. Cost study

Q162. You discover that inspection instructions differ between two production lines. What should be done first?

A. Delay audit
B. Report issue
C. Ignore change
D. Confirm SOP

Q163. What does the QSIT subsystem approach evaluate?

A. Device design
B. Quality subsystems
C. Finance metrics
D. Sales records

Q164. During audit sampling, you find inconsistent supplier approval dates. What should be verified?

A. Risk level
B. Source data
C. Staff role
D. Site policy

Q165. What ensures an audit report is reproducible?

A. Clear evidence

B. Short text
C. Friendly tone
D. Color charts

Q166. A CAPA investigation identifies multiple root causes but no verification plan. What is appropriate?

A. Major NC
B. Minor NC
C. Observation
D. Acceptable

Q167. What does MDSAP use to rate findings?

A. Grading scale
B. Color codes
C. Letter marks
D. Numeric sum

Q168. An auditor observes untrained staff performing product inspection. What is the correct action?

A. Verify records
B. Report finding
C. End audit
D. Ignore claim

Q169. What defines audit consistency across multiple teams?

A. Short reports
B. Faster closure
C. Uniform criteria
D. One auditor

Q170. A supplier's inspection record shows a handwritten correction without signature. What should the auditor record?

A. Minor NC
B. Major NC
C. Observation
D. Acceptable

Q171. What is the auditor's main duty during evidence evaluation?

A. Assess objectivity
B. Record opinions
C. Offer advice
D. Predict trends

Q172. You find two previous CAPAs closed without verification results. What is appropriate action?

A. New finding
B. Observation
C. Skip review
D. Minor note

Q173. During an audit, no evidence is found to verify that supplier evaluations were performed. What should the auditor do?

A. Accept verbal confirmation
B. Record a nonconformance
C. Note as an observation
D. Extend the audit scope

Q174. Auditors note repeated supplier-related deviations over two years. What should be recommended?

A. System audit
B. Supplier removal
C. More samples
D. Ignore trend

Q175. What ensures inspection repeatability?
A. Standard method
B. New staff
C. Faster review
D. Random style

Q176. While reviewing CAPA records, you note only short-term containment actions. What should be reported?
A. Incomplete CAPA
B. Valid CAPA
C. Acceptable CAPA
D. Duplicate CAPA

Q177. What does the QSIT link between subsystems demonstrate?
A. Staff ratio
B. Cost trend
C. Audit time
D. Interdependence

Q178. An auditor finds conflicting design history and validation records. What should be done first?
A. Confirm evidence
B. Write finding
C. Skip review
D. Accept claim

Q179. Which technique best verifies CAPA sustainability?
A. Trend review
B. Peer review
C. Cost check
D. Staff vote

Q180. During MDSAP audit, the team finds similar documentation errors across processes. What should they conclude?
A. Systemic flaw
B. Local issue
C. Minor case
D. Random error

Q181. What verifies a CAPA's long-term success?
A. Shift record
B. Staff feedback
C. Cost review
D. Audit trend

Q182. An auditor notes CAPAs closed quickly with minimal data. What should be concluded?
A. Ineffective process
B. Acceptable speed
C. Corrective success
D. Normal pattern

Q183. Which metric best measures audit program effectiveness?
A. Closure time

B. Audit coverage
C. Staff size
D. Travel budget

Q184. A management review finds recurring issues despite audits. What is implied?
A. Weak CAPA link
B. Excess audits
C. New staff needed
D. Normal variation

Q185. What ensures a CAPA's preventive dimension?
A. Risk control
B. Cost saving
C. Time record
D. Staff count

Q186. During an MDSAP audit, the team identifies overlapping CAPAs. What should be done?
A. Combine causes
B. Split records
C. Close fast
D. Ignore overlap

Q187. What MDSAP task verifies post-market surveillance?
A. Task 7
B. Task 8
C. Task 9
D. Task 10

Q188. An audit reveals incomplete CAPA follow-up actions. What must the auditor record?
A. Major NC
B. Minor NC
C. Observation
D. Acceptable

Q189. What strengthens audit program maturity?
A. Risk ranking
B. Random plan
C. Yearly reuse
D. Minimal scope

Q190. An auditor sees that similar CAPAs recur in calibration control. What conclusion fits best?
A. Systemic issue
B. Random case
C. Isolated event
D. Minor error

Q191. What MDSAP component links design and production controls?
A. Task 4
B. Task 5
C. Task 6
D. Task 7

Q192. A lead auditor finds no CAPA metrics presented to management. What should be reported?
A. Major NC
B. Minor NC
C. Observation
D. Acceptable

Q193. What defines an effective audit cycle?
A. Complete feedback
B. Single audit
C. Quick closure
D. Limited scope
Q194. An auditor notes CAPA records without risk evaluation. What is proper classification?
A. Major NC
B. Minor NC
C. Observation
D. Acceptable
Q195. Which metric indicates CAPA backlog?
A. Open count
B. Cost data
C. Audit days
D. Site visits
Q196. An MDSAP report shows recurring nonconformances in complaint handling. What should management do?
A. Launch CAPA
B. Accept issues
C. Delay action
D. Skip review
Q197. What ensures consistency among multiple auditors?
A. Calibration
B. Rotation
C. Vacation
D. Mentoring
Q198. A follow-up audit finds CAPA evidence incomplete but verified as "closed." What is appropriate?
A. Major NC
B. Observation
C. Acceptable
D. Noted issue
Q199. Which MDSAP task reviews CAPA system?
A. Task 2
B. Task 3
C. Task 4
D. Task 5
Q200. A site's audit schedule excludes one high-risk process. What should be reported?
A. Major NC
B. Minor NC
C. Observation
D. Acceptable

Answer key and Explanation (101-200)

Q101. Answer: C
Explanation: The audit purpose explains why the audit was conducted—its objective and intent. It sets context for evaluating findings and outcomes. Without it, management cannot clearly interpret the audit's goals or the relevance of results.
SubChapter: Audit Report Composition
Q102. Answer: B
Explanation: Conclusions must rest on verifiable evidence, not assumptions. The auditor should gather additional data or documentation before recording a finding to maintain objectivity and factual accuracy.
SubChapter: Evidence Collection Discipline
Q103. Answer: B
Explanation: A system audit assesses the organization's entire quality management system against the ISO 13485 framework. It examines processes collectively to ensure compliance, effectiveness, and regulatory adequacy.
SubChapter: System Auditing Principles
Q104. Answer: B
Explanation: The lead auditor manages the audit process—planning, leading the team, ensuring communication, and finalizing findings. They coordinate resources but do not impose penalties or approve CAPAs.
SubChapter: Audit Leadership Roles
Q105. Answer: C
Explanation: Auditors must support conclusions using evidence and criteria. Calm discussion encourages understanding and allows review of facts without confrontation or compromise of professional integrity.
SubChapter: Dispute Resolution During Closure
Q106. Answer: B
Explanation: MDSAP stands for Medical Device Single Audit Program, a harmonized audit model accepted by multiple regulators (FDA, Health Canada, TGA, ANVISA, PMDA). It consolidates multiple regulatory audits into one process.
SubChapter: MDSAP Overview
Q107. Answer: A
Explanation: Follow-up ensures that corrective actions were effectively implemented and sustained. It confirms that root causes were addressed and recurrence is prevented.
SubChapter: CAPA Verification Process
Q108. Answer: A
Explanation: Significant CAPA delays must be escalated, as they suggest risk of unresolved nonconformities. The auditor's duty is to report, not rewrite or implement the CAPA.
SubChapter: Timeliness in CAPA Follow-Up
Q109. Answer: B
Explanation: Reports must be factual and objective. Auditor opinions introduce subjectivity and bias, undermining the credibility of findings. Reports should rely solely on verifiable evidence.
SubChapter: Audit Report Integrity
Q110. Answer: B
Explanation: MDSAP findings must address all regulatory jurisdictions applicable to the organization. A CAPA must consider each authority's specific requirement to ensure global compliance alignment.
SubChapter: MDSAP Multi-Regulatory Alignment
Q111. Answer: A

Explanation: Findings should be concise, specific, and factual. Clarity prevents misinterpretation and supports precise corrective action by the auditee.
SubChapter: Finding Documentation Standards
Q112. Answer: B
Explanation: The auditor must gather objective evidence—observations, timestamps, or interviews—before classifying the issue. This ensures factual accuracy and defensible reporting.
SubChapter: Objective Evidence Gathering
Q113. Answer: B
Explanation: QSIT (Quality System Inspection Technique) is the FDA's structured approach for inspecting medical device manufacturers to verify compliance with 21 CFR Part 820 requirements.
SubChapter: FDA QSIT Framework
Q114. Answer: B
Explanation: After execution, auditors compile data into a formal report summarizing findings, conclusions, and evidence for management review. Reporting transforms field data into actionable outcomes.
SubChapter: Audit Lifecycle Phases
Q115. Answer: B
Explanation: Verification confirms CAPA effectiveness. Without documented verification, the corrective action process is incomplete and cannot be validated for recurrence prevention.
SubChapter: Effectiveness Verification
Q116. Answer: A
Explanation: Traceability ensures that every finding is directly linked to supporting evidence and the related audit criterion, enabling clear review and regulatory defensibility.
SubChapter: Traceability and Record Control
Q117. Answer: B
Explanation: Repeated findings indicate systemic failures in corrective action management or process control, qualifying as a major system-level deficiency requiring escalation.
SubChapter: Repeat Nonconformance Management
Q118. Answer: B
Explanation: A proper nonconformity statement includes clear objective evidence showing the requirement not met, without assigning blame or speculating about causes.
SubChapter: Nonconformance Documentation
Q119. Answer: B
Explanation: Verbal confirmation cannot replace objective, documented proof. The auditor must record this as incomplete evidence to maintain compliance with verification requirements.
SubChapter: Documentation Verification
Q120. Answer: B
Explanation: Audit success is measured by achievement of defined objectives—comprehensive evaluation, factual reporting, and value-added insight for improvement—not by quantity or speed.
SubChapter: Audit Outcome Evaluation
Q121. Answer: A
Explanation: The scope defines the exact boundaries of an audit—what areas, processes, and periods will be covered. Establishing scope prevents overlap, ensures focus, and clarifies responsibilities for both auditor and auditee throughout the audit lifecycle.
SubChapter: Audit Scope Definition
Q122. Answer: C

Explanation: Auditors should negotiate diplomatically to find a compliant compromise—such as redacted or summary data—while maintaining evidence integrity. Escalation follows only if access refusal prevents objective verification of compliance.
SubChapter: Access and Negotiation Skill

Q123. Answer: B

Explanation: An audit trail provides documented linkage between audit findings, supporting evidence, and applicable criteria. It enables traceability and verification by demonstrating exactly how conclusions were derived from objective data.
SubChapter: Evidence Traceability

Q124. Answer: B

Explanation: Absence of verification documentation means effectiveness cannot be proven. While action occurred, lack of evidence represents a process gap qualifying as a minor nonconformance under ISO 13485 clause 8.5.2 and 8.5.3.
SubChapter: CAPA Verification Control

Q125. Answer: A

Explanation: Accuracy ensures every statement in the audit report precisely reflects verified evidence and correct criteria references. Errors undermine reliability, reduce confidence, and can distort management decisions based on audit outcomes.
SubChapter: Audit Report Integrity

Q126. Answer: C

Explanation: The lead auditor must verify all entries for completeness and factual accuracy before approval. Verification maintains consistency, accountability, and evidentiary strength in the final audit record.
SubChapter: Team Review and Verification

Q127. Answer: A

Explanation: Trend data analysis (e.g., defect rates, deviations) objectively demonstrates whether corrective actions eliminated the root cause and sustained improvement over time, validating CAPA effectiveness.
SubChapter: CAPA Performance Assessment

Q128. Answer: B

Explanation: Contradictory evidence indicates CAPA failure. The auditor must document a new or repeat nonconformance, ensuring management addresses the unresolved issue through renewed investigation and action.
SubChapter: Follow-Up Audit Findings

Q129. Answer: A

Explanation: Specificity makes findings actionable. It clearly states the requirement, evidence, and deviation so the auditee can identify and correct the exact problem without misinterpretation or assumptions.
SubChapter: Finding Writing Skill

Q130. Answer: A

Explanation: Before finalizing a finding, auditors must verify that the skipped step is indeed noncompliant by comparing actual observation to documented procedure. Verification ensures defensible, factual conclusions.
SubChapter: Evidence Verification

Q131. Answer: D

Explanation: The scope outlines coverage and limitations. Including it ensures readers understand which processes were examined and which were excluded, supporting proper interpretation and preventing misuse of results.

SubChapter: Report Structure and Clarity
Q132. Answer: B
Explanation: Lack of root-cause analysis jeopardizes CAPA effectiveness, as symptoms may recur. It represents systemic weakness and qualifies as a major nonconformance per ISO 13485 8.5.2 requirements.
SubChapter: Root-Cause Adequacy
Q133. Answer: A
Explanation: CAPA closure rate, coupled with recurrence data, indicates responsiveness and control of the system. It reflects how efficiently issues are resolved and improvements sustained across reporting periods.
SubChapter: Performance Metrics
Q134. Answer: A
Explanation: Complete documentation is essential for verification. The auditor must request remaining records to ensure evidence sufficiency before forming conclusions about conformity.
SubChapter: Evidence Completeness
Q135. Answer: A
Explanation: Confidential reports must be stored securely with controlled access to authorized personnel only. Protecting sensitive information upholds ethical and regulatory expectations for data integrity.
SubChapter: Confidentiality Control
Q136. Answer: A
Explanation: Preventive actions require documented verification showing how potential issues were mitigated. Without records, the process is noncompliant and must be reported as a nonconformance.
SubChapter: Preventive Action Verification
Q137. Answer: D
Explanation: The fishbone (Ishikawa) diagram helps identify underlying factors contributing to nonconformities by categorizing potential causes under main process elements such as methods, materials, or manpower.
SubChapter: Analytical Techniques for CAPA
Q138. Answer: B
Explanation: Unmonitored CAPAs signal weak management control and risk recurring issues. Prolonged closure time undermines confidence in the CAPA system's responsiveness and regulatory compliance.
SubChapter: Timeliness and Risk Management
Q139. Answer: A
Explanation: Impartiality guarantees all findings—positive or negative—are reported with equal weight. It eliminates favoritism, ensuring balanced representation of facts for objective management decisions.
SubChapter: Fair Presentation Principle
Q140. Answer: B
Explanation: Recurrence across multiple MDSAP tasks indicates a systemic failure affecting several subsystems. Such trends demand higher-level corrective action addressing process or cultural root causes.
SubChapter: Systemic Trend Recognition
Q141. Answer: B
Explanation: An inspection technique refers to a systematic method used to verify conformity, such as sampling, observation, or measurement. Techniques vary by process type and are selected to provide objective, reproducible, and traceable verification results.
SubChapter: Inspection Methodology
Q142. Answer: A

Explanation: Visual inspection confirms label accuracy directly against specifications and approved artwork. It is efficient, objective, and ideal for verifying content, placement, and legibility during quality audits.
SubChapter: Visual Inspection Technique
Q143. Answer: B
Explanation: Sampling enables auditors to evaluate representative evidence when complete inspection is impractical. Properly selected samples provide a statistically valid basis for generalizing conclusions about process compliance and performance.
SubChapter: Sampling Strategy
Q144. Answer: B
Explanation: Systematic sampling uses a fixed interval, such as every 10th item, ensuring even coverage across the population. It offers structure while remaining unbiased when the population order is random.
SubChapter: Sampling Methods
Q145. Answer: A
Explanation: Random sampling gives every item an equal chance of selection, reducing auditor bias and increasing the reliability and fairness of audit conclusions based on evidence.
SubChapter: Unbiased Sampling Technique
Q146. Answer: A
Explanation: Sample failure suggests possible systemic issues. Expanding sample size or audit scope allows confirmation of whether nonconformances are isolated or widespread before reporting final conclusions.
SubChapter: Sample Failure Response
Q147. Answer: C
Explanation: Inspection records provide objective, traceable documentation of test results and observations. They serve as legal and quality evidence demonstrating conformity with specifications and regulatory requirements.
SubChapter: Inspection Documentation
Q148. Answer: B
Explanation: Absence of a defined sampling plan indicates procedural weakness but may not constitute systemic failure. It's a minor nonconformance requiring revision to include statistically sound sampling guidance.
SubChapter: Procedural Compliance
Q149. Answer: A
Explanation: Higher-risk processes require larger or more frequent sampling to ensure adequate evidence for compliance assessment. Risk-based sampling optimizes resources while maintaining reliability and defensibility of audit findings.
SubChapter: Risk-Based Sampling
Q150. Answer: A
Explanation: The auditor must verify why inconsistencies exist by reviewing procedures and interviewing staff before finalizing a finding. Verification prevents misreporting and supports evidence accuracy.
SubChapter: Verification Before Reporting
Q151. Answer: A
Explanation: Consistency ensures different inspectors obtain comparable results under identical conditions. Standardized methods and calibration reduce variability, supporting data reliability and regulatory confidence.
SubChapter: Consistency and Repeatability
Q152. Answer: D

Explanation: The appearance of new defects during reinspection suggests process instability or drift. Investigating potential causes—environmental, procedural, or training-related—helps maintain long-term process control.
SubChapter: Process Stability Evaluation

Q153. Answer: A

Explanation: Inspection objectivity requires judgments based solely on observable, measurable evidence rather than personal opinions or assumptions. This principle ensures consistency and defensibility in audit results.
SubChapter: Objective Evaluation Principle

Q154. Answer: B

Explanation: Before classifying a nonconformance, auditors must verify whether electronic or alternate approvals exist. Verification avoids incorrect conclusions and ensures fair, evidence-based reporting.
SubChapter: Data Verification and Fairness

Q155. Answer: A

Explanation: Checklists structure the inspection process, ensuring consistent focus on critical areas while preventing omissions. They supplement auditor judgment, not replace it.
SubChapter: Checklist Utilization

Q156. Answer: A

Explanation: Over-inspection consumes resources and may not yield proportional benefit. Sampling or statistical inspection provides efficient assurance of quality with less time and cost burden.
SubChapter: Inspection Efficiency

Q157. Answer: A

Explanation: Confidence level increases with sample size. Larger samples reduce uncertainty and better represent the population, improving statistical reliability of audit conclusions.
SubChapter: Sampling Reliability

Q158. Answer: D

Explanation: Identical errors in multiple records suggest a systemic form or template issue, not individual negligence. Auditors should recommend corrective revision of the form or system template.
SubChapter: Systemic Error Recognition

Q159. Answer: A

Explanation: Using a standardized report format ensures findings are organized uniformly across teams, simplifying comparison, review, and trend analysis for management and regulators.
SubChapter: Reporting Standardization

Q160. Answer: A

Explanation: Variation caused by inconsistent checklists indicates lack of harmonization. Leadership must standardize tools and training to align interpretation and ensure uniform assessment across all auditors.
SubChapter: Tool Harmonization and Control

Q161. Answer: A

Explanation: A process-based audit follows the logical flow of an activity—from inputs through outputs—to verify control, effectiveness, and compliance. It focuses on how work is performed and whether it consistently meets defined quality and regulatory standards.
SubChapter: Process-Oriented Auditing

Q162. Answer: D

Explanation: The auditor should verify the approved SOP to determine which instruction version is valid. Comparing observed practices with the documented standard ensures findings are based on objective, factual evidence.
SubChapter: Procedure Verification

Q163. Answer: B

Explanation: QSIT divides the FDA Quality System Regulation into four major subsystems: Management Controls, Design Controls, CAPA, and Production/Process Controls. Inspectors evaluate each to determine the manufacturer's overall compliance and risk level.
SubChapter: FDA QSIT Subsystems

Q164. Answer: B

Explanation: Inconsistent supplier data may arise from documentation errors or outdated files. The auditor should verify original records and databases to confirm validity before classifying the issue as procedural or systemic.
SubChapter: Evidence Verification and Data Validation

Q165. Answer: A

Explanation: A report is reproducible when another qualified auditor could reach the same conclusions using the same evidence and criteria. Clear, detailed documentation ensures objectivity, traceability, and defensibility of findings.
SubChapter: Audit Report Reliability

Q166. Answer: A

Explanation: A CAPA lacking verification cannot prove effectiveness for multiple causes. It represents a serious systemic weakness, requiring classification as a major nonconformance due to incomplete corrective validation.
SubChapter: CAPA Completeness and Verification

Q167. Answer: A

Explanation: The MDSAP grading system evaluates nonconformities on a scale (Grades 1–5) based on severity, frequency, and linkage to requirements. It standardizes interpretation across participating regulatory authorities.
SubChapter: MDSAP Grading System

Q168. Answer: A

Explanation: The auditor must first verify training records to confirm qualification status before concluding a nonconformance. Evidence-based verification ensures fairness and avoids misclassification.
SubChapter: Competence Verification

Q169. Answer: C

Explanation: Applying uniform criteria and procedures ensures consistent conclusions across teams and sites. It minimizes variability and enhances reliability of corporate-level audit data.
SubChapter: Audit Standardization

Q170. Answer: A

Explanation: Unsigned corrections violate data integrity and traceability principles. Although isolated, they represent a procedural lapse that must be corrected through documented control mechanisms.
SubChapter: Data Integrity and Documentation Control

Q171. Answer: A

Explanation: Auditors must evaluate whether evidence is sufficient, reliable, and objective. This judgment determines the strength of findings and supports valid, defensible conclusions.
SubChapter: Evidence Evaluation

Q172. Answer: A

Explanation: Lack of verification indicates ineffective CAPA closure. It must be documented as a new or repeat finding since the organization failed to validate corrective effectiveness.
SubChapter: CAPA Follow-Up Verification

Q173. Answer: B

Explanation: Auditors must rely on objective evidence, not verbal statements. The absence of documented supplier evaluations indicates noncompliance with ISO 13485:2016 requirements for supplier control, warranting a nonconformance.

Q174. Answer: A
Explanation: Repeated supplier nonconformances suggest systemic issues in purchasing controls. Conducting a focused supplier management system audit helps identify root causes and prevent recurrence.
SubChapter: Supplier System Evaluation
Q175. Answer: A
Explanation: Repeatability requires using the same method, environment, and criteria so results remain consistent when rechecked by different inspectors or at different times.
SubChapter: Repeatability and Reliability
Q176. Answer: A
Explanation: Containment actions control immediate issues but don't address root causes. Absence of long-term corrective steps renders the CAPA incomplete, requiring management correction and verification.
SubChapter: CAPA Process Evaluation
Q177. Answer: D
Explanation: QSIT emphasizes how subsystems—CAPA, Management Controls, Design, and Production—interact. Understanding these linkages ensures inspectors assess overall system effectiveness, not isolated processes.
SubChapter: FDA QSIT Integration
Q178. Answer: A
Explanation: Before recording a nonconformance, the auditor must confirm which record set is authoritative. Verification prevents false conclusions and ensures evidence accuracy.
SubChapter: Evidence Validation
Q179. Answer: A
Explanation: Reviewing long-term performance trends—such as defect or complaint rates—validates CAPA sustainability. Declining trend data confirms successful, lasting process improvement.
SubChapter: Long-Term Effectiveness Assessment
Q180. Answer: A
Explanation: Cross-process repetition of documentation errors signals a systemic flaw in document control or training. Auditors should classify it as major, requiring broad corrective action and management review.
SubChapter: Systemic Documentation Review
Q181. Answer: D
Explanation: Trend analysis over time confirms whether implemented actions prevented recurrence. Stable or improved performance data validate that the CAPA effectively addressed the root cause and achieved sustainable process improvement.
SubChapter: CAPA Validation and Monitoring
Q182. Answer: A
Explanation: Rapid closure without supporting data suggests superficial corrections, not root-cause resolution. Effective CAPA requires documented analysis, implementation, and verification of results before closure.
SubChapter: CAPA Process Evaluation
Q183. Answer: B
Explanation: Audit coverage—extent to which critical processes, risks, and sites are assessed—reflects program effectiveness. Comprehensive coverage ensures balanced oversight, risk detection, and continuous quality improvement.
SubChapter: Audit Program Evaluation
Q184. Answer: A

Explanation: Persistent problems after audits indicate weak CAPA linkage between findings and corrective actions. The organization must strengthen feedback loops to ensure audit results drive real improvements.
SubChapter: Audit–CAPA Integration
Q185. Answer: A
Explanation: Preventive actions focus on risk control by identifying and mitigating potential issues before occurrence. Evaluating hazard probability and implementing risk-based actions reduce future nonconformances.
SubChapter: Preventive Action Management
Q186. Answer: A
Explanation: Overlapping CAPAs addressing similar root causes should be consolidated to streamline investigation, eliminate redundancy, and enhance effectiveness monitoring under unified corrective documentation.
SubChapter: MDSAP CAPA Harmonization
Q187. Answer: C
Explanation: Task 9 of MDSAP evaluates post-market surveillance activities, including vigilance, adverse event reporting, and trend analysis, ensuring manufacturers maintain ongoing control of device safety and performance.
SubChapter: MDSAP Task Application
Q188. Answer: A
Explanation: Missing follow-up or verification evidence shows system failure in ensuring effectiveness. It's a major nonconformance that compromises reliability and regulatory compliance of the CAPA process.
SubChapter: CAPA Verification Control
Q189. Answer: A
Explanation: Mature audit programs prioritize based on process risk, frequency, and historical performance. Risk ranking ensures resource focus on high-impact areas, driving improvement and regulatory confidence.
SubChapter: Risk-Based Program Development
Q190. Answer: A
Explanation: Repeated CAPAs within the same process show systemic deficiency, not random error. Root-cause evaluation and management review are required for comprehensive resolution.
SubChapter: Systemic CAPA Analysis
Q191. Answer: B
Explanation: MDSAP Task 5 evaluates Design and Development processes and their integration with Production and Process Controls, ensuring continuity from design intent through manufacturing outcomes.
SubChapter: MDSAP Task Integration
Q192. Answer: B
Explanation: Missing CAPA metrics shows a weakness in performance communication but not necessarily process breakdown. It's a minor nonconformance requiring improvement in management review reporting.
SubChapter: Performance Monitoring and Reporting
Q193. Answer: A
Explanation: An effective cycle includes planning, execution, reporting, corrective action, and follow-up feedback to ensure continuous improvement and system accountability.
SubChapter: Audit Program Lifecycle
Q194. Answer: B

Explanation: Missing risk assessment weakens CAPA prioritization but doesn't always compromise full compliance. It's a minor nonconformance requiring addition of risk evaluation criteria.
SubChapter: Risk-Based CAPA Prioritization

Q195. Answer: A

Explanation: The number of open CAPAs beyond due dates highlights process delays and backlog. Monitoring backlog trends ensures accountability and prompt resolution.
SubChapter: CAPA Timeliness Metric

Q196. Answer: A

Explanation: Recurrence indicates inadequate system control. Management must initiate a CAPA addressing complaint analysis, root cause, and corrective measures to prevent future failures.
SubChapter: Complaint Management and CAPA Linkage

Q197. Answer: A

Explanation: Auditor calibration sessions align understanding of criteria, scoring, and classification standards. This ensures uniform interpretation and consistent reporting across audit teams.
SubChapter: Auditor Calibration

Q198. Answer: A

Explanation: Closing CAPA without full verification evidence violates CAPA control expectations and undermines system credibility. It's a major nonconformance that must be corrected immediately.
SubChapter: Verification and Closure Integrity

Q199. Answer: B

Explanation: MDSAP Task 3 assesses the Corrective and Preventive Action system, verifying processes for investigation, root-cause determination, implementation, and verification of corrective measures.
SubChapter: MDSAP Task Reference

Q200. Answer: A

Explanation: Omitting a high-risk process from audit coverage violates risk-based planning principles. It's a major nonconformance because it compromises audit program completeness and compliance assurance.
SubChapter: Audit Program Risk Planning

Questions (201-300)

Q201. What measures audit team efficiency?

A. On-time finish
B. Evidence ratio
C. Report speed
D. Sample count

Q202. A new auditor struggles to stay on schedule. What should the lead auditor do?

A. Coach directly
B. Replace auditor
C. Shorten scope
D. Skip tasks

Q203. What ensures team coordination during audits?

A. Daily brief
B. Extra forms
C. Silent work
D. Split plans

Q204. Two auditors disagree on evidence interpretation. What should be done?

A. Delay report
B. Choose senior
C. Seek consensus
D. Drop issue

Q205. What defines an audit key performance indicator (KPI)?

A. Quantified measure
B. Auditor opinion
C. Cost estimate
D. Meeting note

Q206. A team finishes fieldwork early but has pending record reviews. What is proper?

A. Continue review
B. Close audit
C. Cut report
D. Cancel review

Q207. Which record proves inspection traceability?

A. Lot sheet
B. Traveler card
C. Log entry
D. Checklist

Q208. During document review, auditors find handwritten inspection notes missing dates. What should be done?

A. Verify records
B. Ignore notes
C. Accept entries
D. Report later

Q209. What maintains inspection record integrity?

A. Secure storage
B. Staff access
C. Color coding
D. Daily copy

Q210. A digital inspection log allows edits without trace. What should be reported?
A. Major NC
B. Minor NC
C. Observation
D. Acceptable
Q211. What strengthens team efficiency during large audits?
A. Long breaks
B. One auditor
C. Less planning
D. Task division
Q212. An audit team member keeps private notes unshared with others. What is best practice?
A. Central sharing
B. Ignore notes
C. Request deletion
D. Accept habit
Q213. Which activity enhances audit performance review?
A. Trend analysis
B. Staff rotation
C. Bonus awards
D. Shorter audits
Q214. Two inspectors use different sampling methods for identical products. What must be done?
A. Standardize method
B. Ignore difference
C. Double sample
D. Shorten test
Q215. What is the first step when auditing inspection records?
A. Count pages
B. Check dates
C. Select forms
D. Define scope
Q216. Audit shows duplicate inspection logs under two managers. What should the auditor conclude?
A. Control gap
B. Good backup
C. Data secure
D. Acceptable
Q217. What tool best measures team communication quality?
A. Feedback form
B. Shift log
C. Expense sheet
D. Checklist
Q218. A follow-up shows inspection logs corrected without justification. What is proper action?
A. Major NC
B. Minor NC
C. Observation
D. Acceptable
Q219. What metric indicates audit resource adequacy?
A. Hours used
B. Cost spent

C. Staff trained
D. Files stored

Q220. Lead auditor notes missing approval signatures on inspection forms. What should be reported?
A. Major NC
B. Minor NC
C. Observation
D. Acceptable

Q221. What ensures audit report consistency across sites?
A. Report template
B. Team rotation
C. Longer audit
D. Local format

Q222. A global company finds regional auditors use different scoring for similar findings. What should management implement?
A. Harmonized scale
B. New auditors
C. Fewer audits
D. Delay reporting

Q223. What improves report readability?
A. Clear structure
B. Long detail
C. Small text
D. Reused notes

Q224. An audit report lacks evidence traceability. What must be corrected?
A. Color charts
B. Extra detail
C. Glossary edit
D. Record linkage

Q225. What MDSAP task validates design controls?
A. Task 5
B. Task 6
C. Task 7
D. Task 8

Q226. A report reviewer finds identical observations repeated from a prior audit. What should be noted?
A. Ineffective CAPA
B. Strong system
C. Faster closure
D. Minimal risk

Q227. What drives continuous audit improvement?
A. Data analysis
B. Short audits
C. New logos
D. Staff rotation

Q228. During MDSAP review, one auditor's grading differs from others. What should be done?
A. Delay closure
B. Ignore grade
C. Report both

D. Team consensus

Q229. What ensures audit follow-up effectiveness?

A. Verified closure
B. Fast approval
C. Short report
D. Lower scope

Q230. A company's internal audit reports lack trend summaries. What should be improved?

A. Data analysis
B. Longer text
C. Faster issue
D. Extra forms

Q231. What demonstrates audit program maturity?

A. Risk-based focus
B. Fixed schedule
C. Equal rotation
D. Minimal reports

Q232. Auditors consistently misclassify observations. What action improves accuracy?

A. Delay review
B. Schedule change
C. Shorter audit
D. Calibration session

Q233. What element enhances management confidence in audits?

A. Reliable data
B. Fast closure
C. Long reports
D. Few findings

Q234. A report summary lists findings but omits recommendations. What should be added?

A. Action guidance
B. More history
C. Less text
D. Extra charts

Q235. What MDSAP task reviews management controls?

A. Task 1
B. Task 2
C. Task 3
D. Task 4

Q236. A CAPA verification shows identical results to the original defect data. What does it indicate?

A. Ineffective CAPA
B. Process stability
C. Full compliance
D. Proper closure

Q237. What tool supports continuous audit learning?

A. Cost tracker
B. Bonus sheet
C. New form
D. Lessons log

Q238. An auditor identifies an outdated SOP still referenced in reports. What is correct?

A. Major NC

B. Minor NC
C. Observation
D. Acceptable

Q239. What reflects audit program improvement over time?
A. Trend reduction
B. More findings
C. Faster audits
D. Fewer forms

Q240. After several MDSAP audits, a company aligns internal and regulatory findings. What does this demonstrate?
A. Program maturity
B. Minimal oversight
C. Random success
D. Data mismatch

Q241. Under 21 CFR Part 820, which element most directly requires manufacturers to maintain procedures for identifying product nonconformities and corrective actions?
A. Design Control
B. CAPA
C. Purchasing Controls
D. Document Control

Q242. Which section of 21 CFR Part 11 defines the criteria for electronic records equivalence to paper records?
A. §11.10
B. §11.30
C. §11.70
D. §11.300

Q243. The primary intent of the FD&C Act Section 501 is to:
A. Define device classification levels
B. Prohibit adulterated devices from interstate commerce
C. Mandate device registration with FDA
D. Regulate post-market advertising

Q244. In EU MDR 2017/745, which Annex specifies requirements for Quality Management Systems of manufacturers?
A. Annex I
B. Annex VII
C. Annex IX
D. Annex X

Q245. ISO 13485:2016 requires risk-based thinking in which activity?
A. Supplier evaluation
B. Design validation
C. Process control planning
D. All the above

Q246. Under 21 CFR Part 820, what is the purpose of management reviews?
A. Assess regulatory changes
B. Evaluate QMS effectiveness and resource needs
C. Perform root-cause analysis
D. Approve product design outputs

Q247. Which regulation requires manufacturers to report adverse events within 30 days to the FDA?

A. 21 CFR 820
B. 21 CFR 803
C. 21 CFR 821
D. 21 CFR 830

Q248. Which best describes the objective of ISO 9001 in medical device contexts?
A. Product safety assurance
B. Customer satisfaction and process improvement
C. Regulatory compliance auditing
D. Design verification documentation

Q249. Under the EU MDR, which actor is responsible for post-market surveillance system implementation?
A. Distributor
B. Manufacturer
C. Competent Authority
D. Notified Body

Q250. What is the primary purpose of device traceability under 21 CFR 821?
A. Facilitate recall and correction actions
B. Support marketing approvals
C. Reduce supplier audits
D. Shorten production cycle time

Q251. Which QSR requirement specifies that document changes must be reviewed and approved by designated personnel?
A. §820.180
B. §820.40
C. §820.90
D. §820.70

Q252. Which of the following best defines Design History File (DHF)?
A. Record of all design outputs
B. Compilation of design and development records showing compliance with plan
C. Device Master Record
D. Supplier audit report

Q253. Which standard defines competence requirements for testing and calibration laboratories used in device manufacture?
A. ISO 17025
B. ISO 13485
C. ISO 14971
D. ISO 9001

Q254. In the FDA QSIT approach, the Design Control subsystem examines:
A. Complaint handling records
B. Supplier qualification procedures
C. Verification of design inputs and outputs
D. Management review minutes

Q255. Which FD&C Act section empowers the FDA to inspect device manufacturing facilities?
A. Section 704
B. Section 510
C. Section 301
D. Section 518

Q256. Under ISO 13485, what is the required output of a management review?

A. Corrective action requests
B. Decisions and actions related to improvement and resource needs
C. Calibration plan
D. Internal audit schedule

Q257. Which post-market activity focuses on analyzing complaint trends to prevent recurrence?
A. CAPA
B. Design Verification
C. Process Validation
D. Internal Audit

Q258. Under EU MDR, a manufacturer's technical documentation must include:
A. Financial statements
B. Advertising materials
C. Design and manufacturing information, risk management, and clinical data
D. Distribution contracts

Q259. The main objective of a Corrective and Preventive Action system is to:
A. Maintain record archives
B. Ensure audit completion
C. Eliminate causes of nonconformities and prevent recurrence
D. Generate supplier performance metrics

Q260. According to ISO 13485, records of training must demonstrate:
A. Budget approval for education
B. Competence to perform assigned tasks
C. Compliance with local labor laws
D. Completion of safety orientation

Q261. Which section of 21 CFR 820 requires verification that purchased products meet specified requirements before use?
A. §820.50
B. §820.30
C. §820.70
D. §820.100

Q262. What is the FDA's intent behind 21 CFR 7 (Subpart C) on Recalls?
A. To penalize manufacturers for device defects
B. To provide guidance for voluntary recalls protecting public health
C. To require mandatory global recalls
D. To document marketing activities

Q263. The FD&C Act Section 510 primarily governs:
A. Premarket approval
B. Establishment registration and device listing
C. Post-market surveillance
D. Inspection enforcement

Q264. According to EU MDR Article 10, manufacturers must implement a QMS that addresses:
A. Design, production, post-market surveillance, and vigilance
B. Financial performance and investor relations
C. Advertising compliance
D. Distributor agreements

Q265. Under ISO 13485, risk management is referenced as a requirement in:
A. Clause 4.2 Documentation
B. Clause 7.1 Planning of product realization

C. Clause 6.2 Human Resources
D. Clause 5.6 Management Review

Q266. 21 CFR 803 requires manufacturers to submit five-day reports when:

A. A death occurs within a hospital setting
B. An event requires immediate corrective action to prevent unreasonable risk to public health
C. The FDA issues a warning letter
D. A customer returns a device for repair

Q267. Which ISO standard details risk management for medical devices?

A. ISO 14971
B. ISO 9001
C. ISO 17025
D. ISO 14001

Q268. The Quality System Inspection Technique (QSIT) identifies how many major subsystems for inspection?

A. Three
B. Four
C. Five
D. Six

Q269. What is the primary purpose of 21 CFR 820.70 – Production and Process Controls?

A. Define supplier selection criteria
B. Ensure manufacturing processes are validated and controlled to consistent specifications
C. Manage device labeling changes
D. Specify employee training records

Q270. Which FD&C Act section authorizes the FDA to require manufacturers to repair, replace, or refund devices posing unreasonable risk?

A. Section 301
B. Section 518
C. Section 510
D. Section 704

Q271. Under EU MDR, a manufacturer's Person Responsible for Regulatory Compliance (PRRC) must:

A. Be based outside the EU
B. Hold a degree in law
C. Possess expertise in QMS and regulatory requirements
D. Be the CEO

Q272. According to ISO 13485, what must be verified before release of product for delivery?

A. Customer complaint closure
B. Conformity to acceptance criteria
C. Supplier qualification approval
D. Budget authorization

Q273. 21 CFR 801 regulates which aspect of medical devices?

A. Labeling and promotional claims
B. Design verification
C. CAPA procedures
D. Training records

Q274. Under ISO 13485, records must be:

A. Retained for ten years after design approval
B. Legible, readily identifiable, and retrievable
C. Stored only electronically

D. Destroyed after five years

Q275. In FDA 21 CFR 806, a manufacturer must report a correction or removal if it:

A. Improves product aesthetics

B. Addresses a violation creating risk to health

C. Is requested by a customer for cost savings

D. Changes packaging design

Q276. Which ISO 13485 clause requires validation of software used in production and service provision?

A. 7.5.6

B. 8.5.1

C. 6.4

D. 5.2

Q277. The primary objective of Post-Market Surveillance (PMS) systems is to:

A. Detect and analyze field performance data to improve device safety and compliance

B. Replace internal audits

C. Eliminate supplier audits

D. Reduce product cost

Q278. According to 21 CFR 820, device master record (DMR) includes:

A. Training certificates

B. Audit reports

C. Specifications and production processes for each device type

D. Financial summaries

Q279. Under ISO 13485, suppliers affecting product quality must be:

A. Certified to ISO 9001

B. Evaluated and selected based on their ability to meet requirements

C. Audited annually by FDA

D. Approved by the notified body

Q280. What is the primary purpose of 21 CFR 830 – Unique Device Identification (UDI)?

A. Simplify marketing applications

B. Provide traceability through device lifecycle for safety and recall management

C. Reduce registration fees

D. Replace serial numbers

Q281. Under 21 CFR 820, which section covers equipment maintenance requirements?

A. §820.70

B. §820.72

C. §820.80

D. §820.90

Q282. What does 21 CFR 4 address for combination products?

A. Labeling

B. Inspections

C. CGMP

D. Audits

Q283. Which clause of ISO 13485 requires identification of training needs?

A. 6.2

B. 7.1

C. 8.1

D. 5.6

Q284. Which FD&C Act section addresses device misbranding?

A. 501
B. 502
C. 510
D. 704

Q285. Which Annex of EU MDR details clinical evaluation requirements?

A. Annex I
B. Annex X
C. Annex IX
D. Annex XII

Q286. Which clause of ISO 13485 requires customer feedback to monitor QMS performance?

A. 7.2.3
B. 8.2.1
C. 8.5.1
D. 6.2.2

Q287. What is the purpose of a Device History Record (DHR)?

A. Design plan
B. Batch record
C. Audit report
D. Budget sheet

Q288. Which authority issues Medical Device Single Audit Program (MDSAP) reports?

A. FDA
B. Competent Authority
C. Notified Body
D. Authorized Auditing Organization

Q289. Under 21 CFR 820, nonconforming product must be:

A. Scrapped
B. Documented
C. Hidden
D. Ignored

Q290. ISO 13485 clause 8.5.2 focuses on:

A. CAPA
B. Audit
C. Complaint
D. Design

Q291. Which FDA program emphasizes top-down inspection focus on management responsibility?

A. QSIT
B. CGMP
C. MDR
D. UDI

Q292. Which document defines device labeling content and placement?

A. DMR
B. DHR
C. CAPA
D. QSP

Q293. Under EU MDR, what must a manufacturer do after serious incident notification?

A. Withdraw CE mark
B. Perform trend analysis
C. Submit FSCA report

D. Notify distributor

Q294. Which ISO 13485 clause requires records of customer property damage?

A. 7.5.10

B. 8.2.4

C. 6.3.1

D. 7.2.2

Q295. 21 CFR 807 requires manufacturers to:

A. Label devices

B. Register facilities

C. Inspect plants

D. Validate designs

Q296. Which ISO standard supports environmental management integration with device production?

A. ISO 9001

B. ISO 14001

C. ISO 17025

D. ISO 14971

Q297. What is the purpose of FDA Form 483?

A. License grant

B. Inspection finding

C. Design approval

D. Risk assessment

Q298. ISO 13485 clause 8.2.4 requires internal audits to be:

A. Continuous

B. Planned

C. Optional

D. Random

Q299. Which FDA regulation addresses device tracking post-distribution?

A. 820

B. 821

C. 803

D. 830

Q300. Under ISO 13485, records of calibration activities must include:

A. Tool age

B. Test dates only

C. Operator opinions

D. Identification of equipment, results, and acceptance criteria

Answer key and Explanation (201-300)

Q201. Answer: A
Explanation: Completing audits within planned timeframes while maintaining evidence quality demonstrates efficient coordination, preparation, and communication among team members. Balanced scheduling ensures productivity without compromising accuracy or thoroughness, supporting continual improvement of audit program performance.
SubChapter: Audit Performance Metrics
Q202. Answer: A
Explanation: The lead auditor should mentor the junior auditor, clarifying expectations and offering guidance to improve effectiveness. Coaching maintains quality standards, supports team growth, and preserves overall audit timing without sacrificing evidence completeness.
SubChapter: Team Leadership and Mentoring
Q203. Answer: A
Explanation: Daily coordination meetings align auditors on progress, findings, and next steps. This communication fosters consistency, avoids overlap, and encourages collaboration, ensuring efficient evidence gathering and cohesive reporting throughout the audit process.
SubChapter: Audit Team Communication
Q204. Answer: C
Explanation: The team should review objective evidence together and compare it with audit criteria to reach agreement. Consensus based on facts—not authority—ensures accuracy, fairness, and alignment with professional auditing standards.
SubChapter: Consensus and Decision-Making
Q205. Answer: A
Explanation: A KPI is a quantifiable measure used to evaluate audit effectiveness, efficiency, or compliance impact—such as on-time completion rate or CAPA closure trend—helping management monitor program health objectively.
SubChapter: Performance Measurement Tools
Q206. Answer: A
Explanation: Finishing early doesn't justify skipping planned reviews. The audit plan must be fully executed to ensure comprehensive coverage, completeness of evidence, and credible conclusions.
SubChapter: Audit Execution Discipline
Q207. Answer: B
Explanation: The traveler card links production steps, inspection data, and responsible personnel for each lot, providing traceability from raw materials to finished product. This ensures accountability and regulatory compliance.
SubChapter: Inspection Record Traceability
Q208. Answer: A
Explanation: The auditor must verify whether date documentation exists elsewhere or was omitted erroneously. Verification before classification prevents inaccurate reporting and maintains evidence integrity.
SubChapter: Record Verification and Validation
Q209. Answer: A
Explanation: Controlled, secure storage protects records from unauthorized alteration or loss, preserving authenticity and traceability. Maintaining proper access controls ensures data reliability for regulatory and quality audits.
SubChapter: Data Security and Integrity
Q210. Answer: A

Explanation: Editable records without audit trails violate data-integrity principles and regulatory standards such as 21 CFR Part 11. It's a major nonconformance requiring immediate correction to ensure secure, traceable data handling.
SubChapter: Electronic Record Control

Q211. Answer: D

Explanation: Dividing tasks by expertise and process area optimizes resources, reduces redundancy, and maintains steady workflow. Clear role assignment ensures every auditor contributes effectively and deadlines are met.
SubChapter: Team Organization and Efficiency

Q212. Answer: A

Explanation: Audit documentation must be transparent within the team. Centralized record sharing ensures completeness, prevents data loss, and allows consistent interpretation of evidence across all members.
SubChapter: Documentation Coordination

Q213. Answer: A

Explanation: Analyzing audit data trends—findings frequency, response time, and closure effectiveness—helps identify systemic issues and drive continuous program improvement.
SubChapter: Performance Review and Improvement

Q214. Answer: A

Explanation: Inconsistent methods compromise comparability of results. Standardizing procedures ensures uniform criteria, reducing variation and supporting reliable conclusions.
SubChapter: Sampling Standardization

Q215. Answer: D

Explanation: Defining the scope identifies which records, timeframes, and processes will be reviewed. Clear scope avoids data overload and directs focus to relevant, risk-based areas.
SubChapter: Audit Preparation for Records

Q216. Answer: A

Explanation: Duplicate uncontrolled logs indicate a documentation-control weakness. They risk conflicting data and loss of record authenticity, requiring corrective action to standardize and centralize record management.
SubChapter: Record Control System Evaluation

Q217. Answer: A

Explanation: Structured feedback from team members after audits evaluates communication effectiveness, identifies barriers, and promotes improved coordination for future engagements.
SubChapter: Communication Assessment

Q218. Answer: B

Explanation: Unauthorized corrections breach documentation protocol but may not indicate intent to falsify. It's a minor nonconformance requiring procedural reinforcement and staff retraining.
SubChapter: Documentation Compliance

Q219. Answer: A

Explanation: Tracking auditor hours against planned effort measures whether sufficient resources were allocated to meet audit objectives, guiding future program planning and scheduling efficiency.
SubChapter: Resource Management Metrics

Q220. Answer: B

Explanation: Missing approvals violate procedural requirements but typically reflect documentation lapses, not systemic failure. It's a minor nonconformance requiring prompt correction and procedural review.
SubChapter: Record Authorization Control

Q221. Answer: A
Explanation: Using standardized report templates aligns structure, terminology, and presentation across sites. It ensures clarity, comparability, and uniform interpretation for management review and regulatory submission, improving corporate audit coherence and oversight efficiency.
SubChapter: Reporting Standardization and Consistency
Q222. Answer: A
Explanation: Variations in scoring undermine comparability and data integrity. Management should implement a harmonized grading scale supported by auditor calibration and training to ensure consistent evaluation across all regions.
SubChapter: Global Audit Alignment
Q223. Answer: A
Explanation: Organized structure with concise headings, consistent formatting, and prioritized findings enhances readability. It enables quick comprehension, facilitates decision-making, and meets both regulatory and management communication needs.
SubChapter: Report Writing Quality
Q224. Answer: D
Explanation: Missing linkage between findings and supporting evidence prevents verification. Reports must clearly reference source records, sample IDs, and observation numbers to ensure traceable, verifiable conclusions.
SubChapter: Evidence Traceability in Reporting
Q225. Answer: A
Explanation: Task 5 of the MDSAP model assesses design and development controls, ensuring devices are designed under controlled processes, validated appropriately, and documented for regulatory compliance and product performance assurance.
SubChapter: MDSAP Design Control Assessment
Q226. Answer: A
Explanation: Repeated findings signal prior corrective actions were ineffective or inadequately verified. The auditor should note systemic CAPA weakness and recommend enhanced root-cause analysis and effectiveness checks.
SubChapter: CAPA Effectiveness and Feedback
Q227. Answer: A
Explanation: Regular analysis of audit outcomes, trends, and metrics identifies strengths and deficiencies. Applying lessons learned supports process refinement, resource optimization, and improved compliance assurance over time.
SubChapter: Continuous Improvement Process
Q228. Answer: D
Explanation: Divergent grading must be resolved by team consensus based on objective evidence and standardized criteria. Alignment ensures regulatory accuracy and uniform data interpretation.
SubChapter: Team Consensus and Grading Calibration
Q229. Answer: A
Explanation: Verified closure confirms that corrective actions are implemented, effective, and sustained. Documented follow-up ensures accountability, preventing recurrence and demonstrating audit program maturity and integrity.
SubChapter: Follow-Up Verification and Closure
Q230. Answer: A
Explanation: Summarizing trends reveals systemic patterns and recurring weaknesses. Including data analysis enhances management insight, promotes proactive improvement, and aligns with ISO 19011 continual-improvement requirements.

SubChapter: Trend Analysis and Reporting Enhancement
Q231. Answer: A
Explanation: Mature programs prioritize audits based on risk, performance, and historical outcomes. This dynamic planning approach maximizes resource use, enhances compliance assurance, and reflects organizational learning capability.
SubChapter: Program Maturity Indicators
Q232. Answer: D
Explanation: Auditor calibration sessions reinforce consistent interpretation of severity, classification, and evidence standards. These sessions ensure reliable, repeatable evaluation across auditors and sites.
SubChapter: Auditor Calibration and Training
Q233. Answer: A
Explanation: Reliable, well-supported audit data builds management trust in conclusions and recommendations. Accuracy and traceability drive actionable decisions and foster organizational credibility during external inspections.
SubChapter: Management Assurance Through Data Integrity
Q234. Answer: A
Explanation: Recommendations translate findings into actionable next steps, guiding corrective and preventive measures. Including them ensures the audit contributes effectively to continual improvement.
SubChapter: Audit Report Enhancement
Q235. Answer: A
Explanation: Task 1 examines management responsibility, review, and resource allocation, ensuring leadership oversight and commitment to regulatory and quality objectives.
SubChapter: MDSAP Management Control Review
Q236. Answer: A
Explanation: Reappearance of the same defects demonstrates CAPA failure. The organization must reassess root-cause analysis and effectiveness verification methods to achieve lasting correction.
SubChapter: CAPA Verification Analysis
Q237. Answer: D
Explanation: Maintaining a lessons-learned log consolidates insights from each audit cycle, helping teams refine methods, avoid past errors, and continuously enhance efficiency and effectiveness.
SubChapter: Knowledge Management in Auditing
Q238. Answer: B
Explanation: Using outdated SOPs shows document-control lapse but not immediate risk if correct procedures exist. It's a minor nonconformance requiring procedural correction and training reinforcement.
SubChapter: Document Control Compliance
Q239. Answer: A
Explanation: A steady reduction in repeated findings and improved closure times indicate a learning system. These trends confirm the audit program's increasing effectiveness and maturity.
SubChapter: Performance Trend Evaluation
Q240. Answer: A
Explanation: Alignment between internal and external audit outcomes shows robust, consistent quality systems and mature audit programs capable of meeting international compliance expectations.
SubChapter: Global Program Integration
Q241. Answer: B
Explanation: CAPA under §820.100 requires manufacturers to investigate nonconformities and implement systemic corrective and preventive actions to eliminate recurrence. Option A relates to

product development; Option C concerns supplier quality; Option D covers record maintenance, not root cause correction.
SubChapter: QSR – CAPA.

Q242. Answer: A

Explanation: Section 11.10 details controls for closed systems, ensuring authenticity, integrity, and confidentiality of electronic records equal to paper versions. Option B addresses open systems, Option C covers signatures and linking, and Option D specifies password security requirements.
SubChapter: FDA CFR Part 11.

Q243. Answer: B

Explanation: Section 501 of the FD&C Act declares that devices not meeting quality or sterility requirements are adulterated and thus unlawful to market. Option A belongs to Section 513; Option C to Section 510; Option D is addressed under 21 CFR 801 Labeling.
SubChapter: FD&C Act Compliance.

Q244. Answer: C

Explanation: Annex IX outlines conformity assessment based on a QMS and technical documentation, forming the core requirement for manufacturers seeking CE marking. Annex I covers general safety, Annex VII addresses notified bodies, and Annex X relates to clinical evaluation.
SubChapter: EU MDR.

Q245. Answer: D

Explanation: ISO 13485 integrates risk-based controls throughout the QMS — in supplier evaluation (§7.4), design validation (§7.3), and process control (§7.5). Every stage demands risk assessment to ensure product safety and effectiveness.
SubChapter: ISO 13485 Risk Management.

Q246. Answer: B

Explanation: Management review (§820.20) requires top management to periodically evaluate the quality system's effectiveness and allocate resources for improvement. Option A is contextual, Option C belongs to CAPA, and Option D falls under design control activities.
SubChapter: QSR – Management Responsibility.

Q247. Answer: B

Explanation: 21 CFR 803 (Medical Device Reporting) mandates submission of adverse event reports within 30 days of awareness. Option A is general QSR; C concerns tracking; D defines UDI system rules.
SubChapter: FDA Reporting and PMS.

Q248. Answer: B

Explanation: ISO 9001 focuses on meeting customer requirements and continuous improvement of process effectiveness. While supportive of medical device quality, it is not device-specific like ISO 13485.
SubChapter: International Standards.

Q249. Answer: B

Explanation: Article 83 assigns the manufacturer responsibility for establishing, documenting, and maintaining a post-market surveillance system. Distributors and notified bodies support but do not own this obligation.
SubChapter: EU MDR – PMS.

Q250. Answer: A

Explanation: 21 CFR 821 ensures manufacturers track certain devices to enable prompt recall or correction in the event of safety issues. It is a public health protection measure, not an efficiency initiative.
SubChapter: FDA Tracking and Recall.

Q251. Answer: B

Explanation: Section 820.40 requires controlled review, approval, and distribution of quality documents to ensure accuracy and prevent use of obsolete versions. §820.180 covers record retention; §820.90 addresses nonconforming product; §820.70 refers to production controls.
SubChapter: QSR Documentation.
Q252. Answer: B
Explanation: Per §820.30 (j), the DHF contains records demonstrating that design was developed according to the approved plan and requirements. It differs from the DMR, which details manufacturing specifications.
SubChapter: Design Control.
Q253. Answer: A
Explanation: ISO/IEC 17025 specifies competence for laboratories performing tests and calibrations, ensuring valid results for device verification. 13485 and 9001 are QMS standards; 14971 covers risk management.
SubChapter: International Standards – Testing Competence.
Q254. Answer: C
Explanation: QSIT design controls focus on verifying that design inputs meet outputs and changes are controlled before release. Options A and B belong to other subsystems; D is management responsibility.
SubChapter: FDA QSIT.
Q255. Answer: A
Explanation: Section 704 grants the FDA authority to enter and inspect facilities where regulated devices are manufactured to ensure compliance with the Act. §510 covers registration, §301 lists prohibitions, and §518 addresses remedies.
SubChapter: FD&C Act – Inspections.
Q256. Answer: B
Explanation: Clause 5.6 mandates management reviews to produce documented decisions regarding improvements, QMS changes, and resource allocations. Other options may result indirectly but are not explicit outputs.
SubChapter: ISO 13485 – Management Review.
Q257. Answer: A
Explanation: CAPA processes analyze complaint data to identify systemic issues and prevent recurrence. Design verification validates outputs; process validation confirms production capability; audits evaluate QMS compliance.
SubChapter: PMS – CAPA Integration.
Q258. Answer: C
Explanation: Annex II and III require comprehensive technical documentation including design details, risk management, and clinical evaluation to demonstrate conformity. Options A, B, and D are non-technical records.
SubChapter: EU MDR – Documentation.
Q259. Answer: C
Explanation: CAPA systems identify and eliminate root causes of quality problems to prevent recurrence, strengthening process control and compliance. Other options are supporting activities, not primary objectives.
SubChapter: QSR – CAPA.
Q260. Answer: B
Explanation: Clause 6.2 requires evidence that personnel are competent based on education, training, skills, and experience. It emphasizes competence, not attendance or budget.
SubChapter: ISO 13485 – Personnel Competence.
Q261. Answer: A

Explanation: Section 820.50 covers Purchasing Controls, requiring manufacturers to establish procedures ensuring suppliers and purchased products conform to specifications. Options B and C concern design and production; D is CAPA-related.
SubChapter: QSR – Purchasing Controls.

Q262. Answer: B

Explanation: 21 CFR 7 guides voluntary recalls, outlining notification, effectiveness checks, and termination to protect public health. It's not punitive or globally binding.
SubChapter: FDA CFR – Recalls.

Q263. Answer: B

Explanation: Section 510 requires establishments to register annually and list devices marketed in the U.S., forming the FDA's inventory of regulated manufacturers. Other sections cover approval (515) and inspection (704).
SubChapter: FD&C Act – Registration.

Q264. Answer: A

Explanation: Article 10 requires a comprehensive QMS covering design, manufacture, final inspection, PMS, and vigilance. The QMS must align with Annex IX for conformity assessment.
SubChapter: EU MDR – QMS Integration.

Q265. Answer: B

Explanation: Clause 7.1 requires manufacturers to apply risk management in planning product realization. Risk must be considered from design through delivery. Other clauses address documentation, personnel, or review.
SubChapter: ISO 13485 – Risk Integration.

Q266. Answer: B

Explanation: A five-day report is mandatory when FDA requests it or when events necessitate urgent correction to mitigate public risk. Routine repairs don't qualify.
SubChapter: FDA CFR – MDR.

Q267. Answer: A

Explanation: ISO 14971 specifies a structured process for risk analysis, evaluation, control, and monitoring through a device's lifecycle. Other standards focus on quality systems or environmental management.
SubChapter: Risk Management Standards.

Q268. Answer: B

Explanation: QSIT organizes FDA inspections around four subsystems: Management Controls, Design Controls, CAPA, and Production and Process Controls. Each subsystem provides structured focus for compliance audits.
SubChapter: FDA QSIT.

Q269. Answer: B

Explanation: §820.70 mandates control and validation of production processes to guarantee product conformance. Supplier and training requirements are covered elsewhere in the QSR.
SubChapter: QSR – Process Controls.

Q270. Answer: B

Explanation: Section 518 permits FDA to issue remedial orders such as repairs or refunds for devices presenting serious risk. Other sections cover prohibited acts, registration, and inspection.
SubChapter: FD&C Act – Remedies.

Q271. Answer: C

Explanation: Article 15 requires manufacturers to appoint a qualified PRRC experienced in QMS and device regulations. This role ensures ongoing compliance and vigilance reporting.
SubChapter: EU MDR – Governance.

Q272. Answer: B
Explanation: Clause 8.2.6 requires verification that product meets defined acceptance criteria before release, ensuring traceable evidence of conformity.
SubChapter: ISO 13485 – Product Release.
Q273. Answer: A
Explanation: Part 801 defines labeling requirements, ensuring information is accurate and not misleading. Design and CAPA belong to Part 820.
SubChapter: FDA CFR – Labeling.
Q274. Answer: B
Explanation: Clause 4.2.5 requires records to remain legible, identifiable, and retrievable for traceability and regulatory review. Retention time is defined by regulation or contract, not fixed.
SubChapter: Documentation Control.
Q275. Answer: B
Explanation: Part 806 requires reporting of corrections or removals to remedy violations that may pose risk to health. Cosmetic or economic changes are exempt.
SubChapter: FDA CFR – Corrections and Removals.
Q276. Answer: A
Explanation: Clause 7.5.6 mandates software validation when used in production or service to ensure it meets intended purpose. Other clauses address resources, customer focus, and improvement.
SubChapter: ISO 13485 – Software Validation.
Q277. Answer: A
Explanation: PMS collects and analyzes real-world data to detect safety signals and drive preventive actions for continuous compliance with regulatory expectations.
SubChapter: PMS – Data Analysis.
Q278. Answer: C
Explanation: §820.181 requires the DMR to contain device specifications, production methods, quality assurance procedures, and packaging specifications to ensure consistent manufacture.
SubChapter: QSR – DMR Control.
Q279. Answer: B
Explanation: Clause 7.4 requires evaluation and selection of suppliers based on their capability to meet specified requirements affecting product quality. Certification is optional, not mandatory.
SubChapter: Supplier Quality.
Q280. Answer: B
Explanation: UDI ensures each device has a unique identifier for tracking, recall, and adverse event analysis, enhancing patient safety and regulatory oversight.
SubChapter: FDA CFR – UDI System.
Q281. Answer: B
Explanation: Section 820.72 requires calibration and maintenance of inspection and test equipment to assure accuracy and precision of measurements. Other sections address process control, receiving acceptance, and nonconformance handling.
SubChapter: QSR – Equipment Control.
Q282. Answer: C
Explanation: Part 4 details Current Good Manufacturing Practice requirements for combination products containing device and drug components, ensuring compliance with both 21 CFR 210/211 and 820. Other options focus on specific subsystems not covered by Part 4.
SubChapter: FDA CFR – CGMP Integration.
Q283. Answer: A

Explanation: Clause 6.2 requires organizations to identify training needs and ensure competence of personnel affecting product quality. Other clauses cover planning, measurement, and review activities.
SubChapter: ISO 13485 – Competence.

Q284. Answer: B

Explanation: Section 502 defines misbranding conditions such as false or misleading labeling, ensuring accuracy and honesty in communication. Section 501 concerns adulteration; 510 and 704 cover registration and inspection.
SubChapter: FD&C Act – Labeling.

Q285. Answer: B

Explanation: Annex X of EU MDR 2017/745 defines clinical evaluation and performance studies required for CE marking. Annex I covers safety requirements; Annex IX addresses QMS conformity; Annex XII concerns certificates.
SubChapter: EU MDR – Clinical Evaluation.

Q286. Answer: B

Explanation: Clause 8.2.1 mandates collection and analysis of customer feedback to assess QMS effectiveness. It forms part of the measurement and analysis process.
SubChapter: ISO 13485 – Feedback.

Q287. Answer: B

Explanation: A DHR contains production history for each batch to verify that manufacturing followed approved procedures and specifications. Other options relate to planning or administration.
SubChapter: QSR – Records.

Q288. Answer: D

Explanation: MDSAP audits are performed by authorized Auditing Organizations recognized by participating regulators (FDA, Health Canada, TGA, etc.). They issue reports accepted across jurisdictions.
SubChapter: International Regulation.

Q289. Answer: B

Explanation: Section 820.90 requires documentation and evaluation of nonconforming product to determine disposition and corrective action. Scrapping may occur later, but recording is mandatory.
SubChapter: QSR – Nonconformance.

Q290. Answer: A

Explanation: Clause 8.5.2 covers Corrective Action, requiring analysis of nonconformities to eliminate causes and prevent recurrence. Audit and complaint controls are handled elsewhere.
SubChapter: ISO 13485 – CAPA.

Q291. Answer: A

Explanation: QSIT begins inspections with management controls to assess QMS effectiveness and commitment, ensuring oversight of all subsystems. Other programs are complementary tools.
SubChapter: FDA Inspection Systems.

Q292. Answer: A

Explanation: The Device Master Record (DMR) includes approved labeling content and placement instructions to ensure consistency and regulatory compliance. Other documents record execution or procedures.
SubChapter: QSR – DMR.

Q293. Answer: C

Explanation: Manufacturers must submit a Field Safety Corrective Action (FSCA) report and Field Safety Notice to competent authorities and users after serious incidents. Other actions may follow based on risk.
SubChapter: EU MDR – Vigilance.

Q294. Answer: A

Explanation: Clause 7.5.10 mandates records if customer property is lost, damaged, or otherwise unsuitable for use, ensuring accountability and communication. Other clauses cover different quality functions.
SubChapter: ISO 13485 – Customer Property.

Q295. Answer: B

Explanation: Part 807 covers establishment registration and device listing, helping FDA maintain manufacturer records for oversight and inspection purposes.
SubChapter: FDA CFR – Registration.

Q296. Answer: B

Explanation: ISO 14001 addresses environmental management systems, helping organizations control environmental aspects within regulated industries like medical devices. It complements QMS standards but is not mandatory for certification.
SubChapter: Environmental Standards.

Q297. Answer: B

Explanation: Form 483 lists observations made by FDA inspectors indicating noncompliance with CGMP or QSR requirements. It serves as official communication to management for correction.
SubChapter: FDA Compliance Enforcement.

Q298. Answer: B

Explanation: Clause 8.2.4 requires organizations to plan internal audits at defined intervals to determine QMS conformance and effectiveness. Random audits may supplement but planning is mandatory.
SubChapter: ISO 13485 – Audits.

Q299. Answer: B

Explanation: 21 CFR 821 requires manufacturers to track specific devices post-distribution to facilitate recall and field correction. Other parts cover QSR, reporting, and UDI.
SubChapter: FDA Tracking.

Q300. Answer: D

Explanation: Clause 7.6 requires records to identify equipment, calibration results, and acceptance criteria to ensure measurement accuracy. Incomplete records invalidate data integrity.
SubChapter: ISO 13485 – Calibration.

Questions (301-400)

Q301. Which regulation defines requirements for medical device labeling?

A. 21 CFR 801
B. 21 CFR 820
C. 21 CFR 821
D. 21 CFR 830

Q302. What is the primary goal of CAPA under QSR?

A. Eliminate root causes
B. Track supplier data
C. Improve design layout
D. Monitor production flow

Q303. Under ISO 13485, what should management reviews determine?

A. Marketing goals
B. Resource needs
C. Supplier pricing
D. Advertising cost

Q304. What is the function of a Device Master Record (DMR)?

A. Production blueprint
B. Cost ledger
C. Audit checklist
D. Training log

Q305. Which ISO 13485 clause covers control of monitoring and measuring equipment?

A. 7.6
B. 8.2
C. 6.3
D. 5.2

Q306. Under 21 CFR 803, which report must be filed for an event causing serious injury?

A. 483 Form
B. MDR
C. FSCA
D. QAR

Q307. Which document defines manufacturing process validation activities?

A. Quality Plan
B. Validation Protocol
C. CAPA Log
D. Training Matrix

Q308. Under EU MDR, which article mandates unique device identification?

A. 24
B. 27
C. 29
D. 32

Q309. Which FD&C Act section defines prohibited acts related to adulteration or misbranding?

A. 301
B. 502
C. 510
D. 704

Q310. What is the purpose of ISO 13485 clause 8.3?

A. Control of nonconforming product
B. Document management
C. Supplier evaluation
D. Training review

Q311. Which agency coordinates the Medical Device Single Audit Program (MDSAP)?

A. IMDRF
B. WHO
C. EMA
D. USP

Q312. Under 21 CFR 820, which section covers process validation requirements?

A. 820.75
B. 820.30
C. 820.50
D. 820.90

Q313. What does ISO 13485 clause 8.5.3 specify?

A. Training needs
B. Design change
C. Preventive action
D. Audit plan

Q314. Which document lists approved suppliers and their evaluation results?

A. Approved Vendor List
B. Audit Plan
C. Quality Manual
D. Device History Record

Q315. Which FDA regulation defines requirements for device corrections and removals?

A. 803
B. 806
C. 807
D. 820

Q316. What is the role of internal audits under ISO 13485?

A. Verify QMS conformity
B. Approve designs
C. Record complaints
D. Train staff

Q317. What is required under 21 CFR 820.20 for top management?

A. QMS oversight
B. Supplier selection
C. Product labeling
D. Complaint review

Q318. What is the key requirement of EU MDR Article 83?

A. Post-market surveillance system
B. Clinical trial registration
C. CE mark renewal
D. Distributor approval

Q319. What does ISO 13485 clause 7.3 cover?

A. Process validation
B. Purchasing controls
C. Customer feedback

D. Design and development

Q320. Under FD&C Act Section 704, the FDA may:

A. Inspect facilities

B. Set prices

C. Approve patents

D. License distributors

Q321. During a supplier audit, you find calibration records missing for test equipment. Which QSR section applies?

A. §820.72

B. §820.70

C. §820.30

D. §820.90

Q322. A company uses an electronic document control system. What must it ensure under 21 CFR Part 11?

A. User authentication

B. Supplier approval

C. Design review

D. CAPA entry

Q323. Scenario: A manufacturer receives complaints of devices failing after sterilization. Investigation reveals inadequate temperature validation. What process was violated?

A. Design input

B. Process validation

C. Document control

D. Supplier evaluation

Q324. Which ISO 13485 clause addresses customer communication?

A. 7.2.3

B. 7.3.5

C. 8.3.1

D. 5.4.2

Q325. Scenario: During inspection, an FDA investigator asks for the CAPA log. What should it demonstrate?

A. Resource spending

B. Issue trends

C. Root cause elimination

D. Staff promotions

Q326. What is the role of management representative under ISO 13485?

A. Implement and maintain QMS

B. Approve purchase orders

C. File patent applications

D. Create marketing plans

Q327. Scenario: An EU manufacturer discovers its post-market data show higher incident rates. What is the correct action under Article 83?

A. Modify PMS plan

B. Report to CEO

C. Stop distribution

D. Archive records

Q328. Which FD&C Act section gives FDA authority to seize adulterated devices?

A. 518

B. 301
C. 510
D. 304

Q329. Under ISO 13485, design transfer ensures:
A. Smooth shift from development to production
B. Supplier approval
C. Audit preparation
D. Complaint review

Q330. Scenario: An FDA inspector observes that design verification results lack objective evidence. Which violation applies?
A. §820.30(f)
B. §820.50
C. §820.90
D. §820.72

Q331. Under EU MDR, what is the purpose of vigilance reporting?
A. Document financial results
B. Notify serious incidents
C. Register product models
D. Evaluate suppliers

Q332. ISO 13485 clause 8.5.2 requires organizations to:
A. Correct nonconformities
B. Manage suppliers
C. Approve labels
D. Validate software

Q333. Scenario: A manufacturer changes a critical design element without documentation. What clause is violated?
A. 7.3.9
B. 6.2.1
C. 8.2.3
D. 5.6.2

Q334. What is required by 21 CFR 820.198?
A. Complaint handling
B. CAPA documentation
C. Supplier audit
D. Label verification

Q335. Which clause of ISO 13485 requires control of outsourced processes?
A. 4.1
B. 7.5
C. 8.1
D. 6.4

Q336. Scenario: A supplier changes raw material composition affecting device performance. What must the manufacturer do first?
A. Replace personnel
B. File patent update
C. Halt all shipments
D. Evaluate change impact

Q337. Under ISO 13485, clause 8.4 requires evaluation of:
A. Supplier data

B. Market feedback
C. Nonconformance rate
D. Outsourced processes

Q338. Which part of 21 CFR defines device tracking requirements?
A. 820
B. 821
C. 803
D. 807

Q339. Scenario: An EU manufacturer receives notice that its notified body certificate will expire soon. What must it do?
A. Renew CE marking
B. Suspend production
C. File MDR report
D. Change PRRC

Q340. According to ISO 13485, clause 7.4.3 requires purchasing data to include:
A. Product specifications
B. Tax details
C. Employee names
D. Marketing codes

Q341. What is the purpose of ISO 13485 clause 7.5.9 on traceability?
A. Identify product status
B. Track production costs
C. Measure staff output
D. Manage budgets

Q342. Which CFR section mandates establishment registration before device distribution?
A. 21 CFR 807
B. 21 CFR 803
C. 21 CFR 806
D. 21 CFR 821

Q343. Scenario: A design engineer updates risk analysis documents after field failures. Which ISO 13485 clause applies?
A. 7.1
B. 7.3.9
C. 8.2.2
D. 5.6

Q344. Under EU MDR, which Annex outlines post-market surveillance plan contents?
A. Annex III
B. Annex IX
C. Annex X
D. Annex XI

Q345. Which FD&C Act section authorizes injunctions against violating firms?
A. 302
B. 304
C. 510
D. 518

Q346. Scenario: An internal audit reveals employees not trained on revised SOPs. Which ISO 13485 clause is violated?
A. 6.2

B. 7.4
C. 8.2
D. 5.5

Q347. Under 21 CFR 820.40, document approval must be:
A. Delegated externally
B. Oral, informal, quick
C. Untracked, flexible
D. Reviewed, signed, dated

Q348. What is the intent of ISO 13485 clause 8.2.3 on monitoring?
A. Evaluate process conformity
B. Measure profit margin
C. Review supplier budgets
D. Track marketing success

Q349. Scenario: After an FDA inspection, a warning letter cites incomplete validation records. What should management do first?
A. Submit CAPA plan
B. Terminate staff
C. File complaint
D. Delay response

Q350. Which ISO 13485 clause requires control of environmental conditions?
A. 6.4
B. 7.2
C. 8.3
D. 5.5

Q351. Under EU MDR, which article describes general obligations of manufacturers?
A. 10
B. 15
C. 27
D. 56

Q352. Scenario: A device component supplier loses ISO 13485 certification. What must the manufacturer do?
A. Suspend audits
B. Ignore situation
C. Reevaluate supplier
D. Replace auditor

Q353. Which 21 CFR part governs unique identification labeling?
A. 801
B. 830
C. 821
D. 807

Q354. What is the role of preventive maintenance records?
A. Prove equipment reliability
B. Track device failures
C. Manage supplier lists
D. Plan audit schedules

Q355. Scenario: Complaint trending identifies repeat software malfunctions. What is the next regulatory step?
A. Initiate CAPA

B. Notify HR
C. Close complaint
D. File invoice

Q356. ISO 13485 clause 7.3.5 requires design reviews to be:
A. Systematic and recorded
B. Informal and verbal
C. Optional and rare
D. Confidential only

Q357. Which FD&C Act section grants FDA authority to require premarket approval?
A. 515
B. 510
C. 501
D. 518

Q358. Scenario: An EU distributor reports counterfeit devices in circulation. What is the manufacturer's duty?
A. Recall staff
B. Halt production
C. Ignore issue
D. Notify authorities

Q359. Under ISO 13485 clause 8.5.1, improvement must be:
A. Planned and documented
B. Random and informal
C. Delayed and reactive
D. Verbal and unrecorded

Q360. Scenario: During validation, temperature sensors show inconsistent readings. What must be done first?
A. Investigate instruments
B. Redo audit
C. File MDR
D. Stop labeling

Q361. Which section of 21 CFR 820 covers design validation?
A. 820.30 (g)
B. 820.70 (b)
C. 820.90 (a)
D. 820.100 (b)

Q362. Under ISO 13485, what does clause 4.2.1 require?
A. Audit plan
B. Risk matrix
C. QMS documentation
D. Marketing file

Q363. Scenario: An internal audit identifies incomplete CAPA verification. What must be done first?
A. Review effectiveness
B. Close record
C. Escalate to HR
D. Pause production

Q364. What is the objective of ISO 13485 clause 5.3 on quality policy?
A. Guide QMS direction
B. Set audit schedule

C. Define sales targets
D. List training hours
Q365. Scenario: An EU MDR audit finds missing PSUR updates. Which article is violated?
A. 86
B. 83
C. 91
D. 27
Q366. Under 21 CFR 820.180, which records are exempt from routine FDA inspection?
A. Device master record
B. Complaint files
C. Supplier audits
D. Management review
Q367. Scenario: A production line change affects sterilization parameters. What action is mandatory?
A. Revalidation
B. Price review
C. Audit delay
D. Staff transfer
Q368. Which FD&C Act section covers banned devices?
A. 516
B. 510
C. 704
D. 301
Q369. Under ISO 13485, clause 7.5.3.2 requires identification of:
A. Product status
B. Audit scope
C. Supplier names
D. Budget codes
Q370. Scenario: A CAPA team closes a record without verifying effectiveness. During audit, repeat issues occur. What is the root problem?
A. Late shipment
B. Incorrect budget
C. Poor HR training
D. Ineffective verification
Q371. Which EU MDR Annex details quality management system requirements for conformity assessment?
A. Annex IX
B. Annex X
C. Annex XI
D. Annex XII
Q372. Under 21 CFR 820.22, internal audits must be:
A. Planned and periodic
B. Random and informal
C. Optional and rare
D. Delegated externally
Q373. Scenario: Supplier complaints show consistent spec failures. Which clause requires supplier reevaluation?
A. 7.4.1
B. 8.5.2

C. 6.2.2
D. 5.3.1
Q374. Which CFR part addresses foreign manufacturer registration?
A. 821 Subpart C
B. 820 Subpart E
C. 803 Subpart D
D. 807 Subpart B
Q375. Scenario: An engineer uses unapproved software for testing devices. Which regulation is violated?
A. 820.70 (i)
B. 820.30 (g)
C. 820.90 (b)
D. 820.120 (a)
Q376. Which ISO 13485 clause addresses risk management throughout product realization?
A. 7.1
B. 6.3
C. 5.6
D. 8.2
Q377. Scenario: Complaint investigation finds label mix-up causing wrong dosage. Which section applies?
A. 820.120
B. 820.70
C. 820.50
D. 820.180
Q378. Which FD&C Act section authorizes records inspection?
A. 516
B. 510
C. 518
D. 704
Q379. Scenario: A design team fails to document input requirements. Which clause is breached?
A. 7.3.2
B. 7.5.3
C. 8.3.4
D. 5.5.2
Q380. According to 21 CFR 820.25, training must be:
A. Documented and effective
B. Casual and optional
C. Annual and untracked
D. Delegated to auditors
Q381. Digital QMS platforms implementing e-signatures must comply with which FDA rule?
A. 21 CFR Part 11
B. 21 CFR Part 820
C. 21 CFR Part 801
D. 21 CFR Part 830
Q382. Scenario: A manufacturer integrates AI-based image analysis in device design. Which ISO 13485 clause ensures risk management throughout the lifecycle?
A. 7.1
B. 8.5

C. 4.2
D. 6.3
Q383. Which EU MDR article defines obligations for importers verifying CE conformity?
A. Article 27
B. Article 10
C. Article 13
D. Article 86
Q384. Cloud-based complaint management systems must ensure data:
A. Integrity and auditability
B. Portability only
C. Simplicity only
D. Confidentiality ignored
Q385. Scenario: A supplier uses blockchain for device component traceability. Which requirement must still be met?
A. Data validation
B. Manual logging
C. Visual labels
D. Physical forms
Q386. Which FD&C Act section enables FDA to mandate postmarket surveillance studies?
A. 522
B. 515
C. 518
D. 704
Q387. Scenario: During MDSAP audit, the team requests evidence of data integrity across digital CAPA workflows. What documentation is reviewed?
A. Marketing flyers
B. Expense reports
C. Shipping invoices
D. Audit trail logs
Q388. ISO 13485 requires calibration records to include:
A. Results, equipment ID, and acceptance criteria
B. Operator name only
C. Cost of testing
D. Date alone
Q389. Which EU MDR Annex describes technical documentation content for conformity?
A. Annex II
B. Annex IX
C. Annex X
D. Annex XI
Q390. Scenario: A mobile app update modifies device control functions. Which regulatory requirement applies?
A. Design change evaluation
B. Marketing reapproval
C. Label redesign
D. Distributor audit
Q391. Under ISO 13485, what does clause 7.5.7 require for sterile devices?
A. Label font check
B. Routine color inspection

C. Warranty record review
D. Controlled environment validation

Q392. FDA 21 CFR 803 requires MDR submissions in which format?
A. Electronic eMDR
B. Printed paper only
C. Fax confirmation
D. Verbal notification

Q393. Scenario: A manufacturer integrates predictive analytics in PMS to detect early trends. Which ISO 13485 clause supports this?
A. 8.4
B. 7.2
C. 6.4
D. 4.3

Q394. Which FD&C Act section authorizes FDA to issue warning letters before enforcement?
A. 305
B. 510
C. 704
D. 518

Q395. Scenario: A cloud-based QMS is hosted offshore. What must the manufacturer ensure?
A. Access restriction to users
B. Encryption removal
C. Server anonymity
D. Data access for regulatory inspection

Q396. ISO 13485 clause 8.5.2 emphasizes what activity before CAPA closure?
A. Effectiveness verification
B. Marketing approval
C. Legal consultation
D. Cost accounting

Q397. Under EU MDR, which article mandates transparency via EUDAMED database?
A. Article 33
B. Article 10
C. Article 86
D. Article 13

Q398. Scenario: FDA requests device traceability data within 48 hours. Which system should supply this?
A. UDI and DHR
B. CRM and ERP
C. HR and Payroll
D. SCM and Finance

Q399. ISO 13485 clause 8.2.1 emphasizes feedback analysis for:
A. Employee reward calculation
B. Product marketing and advertising
C. QMS improvement and risk reduction
D. Financial planning

Q400. Scenario: An IVD manufacturer adopts cloud-based performance monitoring. Which EU IVDR requirement applies?
A. Continuous performance evaluation
B. Label font verification

C. Distributor pricing control
D. Advertising approval

Answer key and Explanation (301-400)

Q301. Answer: A
Explanation: Part 801 defines labeling standards ensuring information accuracy, clarity, and non-misleading claims. It governs both device labels and user instructions. Other parts address quality systems, tracking, and identification systems. SubChapter: FDA CFR – Labeling.
Q302. Answer: A
Explanation: CAPA aims to identify and eliminate root causes of nonconformities and prevent recurrence. It integrates complaint data, audit results, and trend analysis to enhance process control. Other actions support broader quality efforts but not the core CAPA objective. SubChapter: QSR – CAPA.
Q303. Answer: B
Explanation: Clause 5.6 requires management to assess QMS performance and determine resource needs for improvement. Reviews evaluate feedback, audit results, and corrective actions, driving continuous improvement of system effectiveness. Other items are not part of formal management review content. SubChapter: ISO 13485 – Management Review.
Q304. Answer: A
Explanation: The DMR provides the complete blueprint for device manufacture, including specifications, processes, and inspection procedures. It ensures each product is made consistently to approved standards, enabling traceability and compliance with 21 CFR 820.181. SubChapter: QSR – Documentation.
Q305. Answer: A
Explanation: Clause 7.6 requires control, calibration, and maintenance of measuring equipment to ensure valid results. Devices must be traceable to recognized standards and verified after repair. Uncontrolled instruments may compromise product quality and compliance. SubChapter: ISO 13485 – Equipment Control.
Q306. Answer: B
Explanation: The Medical Device Report (MDR) is required for incidents resulting in death, serious injury, or malfunction that could cause harm. Manufacturers must submit within 30 days of awareness. Other documents serve unrelated regulatory or audit purposes. SubChapter: FDA CFR – Reporting.
Q307. Answer: B
Explanation: Validation Protocols describe objectives, responsibilities, acceptance criteria, and test procedures for process validation, ensuring consistent product quality. They must be approved before execution and archived in compliance records. Other documents provide support but not core validation structure. SubChapter: QSR – Validation.
Q308. Answer: B
Explanation: Article 27 introduces the Unique Device Identification (UDI) system to enhance traceability and recall management. It applies across all device classes and aligns with 21 CFR 830 requirements for global harmonization. SubChapter: EU MDR – UDI.
Q309. Answer: A
Explanation: Section 301 prohibits the introduction, sale, or distribution of adulterated or misbranded medical devices. It forms the foundation for enforcement actions such as warning letters and seizures. Other sections address labeling, registration, or inspections. SubChapter: FD&C Act – Compliance.
Q310. Answer: A
Explanation: Clause 8.3 specifies control of nonconforming product to prevent unintended use or delivery. Actions include segregation, documentation, and disposition, ensuring traceability and corrective follow-up. It's a core preventive safeguard in QMS. SubChapter: ISO 13485 – Nonconformance.
Q311. Answer: A

Explanation: The International Medical Device Regulators Forum (IMDRF) oversees MDSAP, enabling one audit recognized by multiple regulatory authorities like FDA, Health Canada, and TGA. It enhances efficiency while maintaining robust oversight. SubChapter: Global Regulatory Programs.

Q312. Answer: A

Explanation: Section 820.75 requires validation of processes where output cannot be fully verified by inspection or testing. Validation must prove consistent conformity. Other sections concern design, purchasing, and nonconformance. SubChapter: QSR – Validation.

Q313. Answer: C

Explanation: Clause 8.5.3 mandates preventive actions to eliminate potential nonconformities before occurrence. Organizations must analyze trends and risk data to identify opportunities for prevention. Other activities are handled under different clauses. SubChapter: ISO 13485 – Preventive Action.

Q314. Answer: A

Explanation: The Approved Vendor List (AVL) maintains records of supplier qualification, performance, and approval status, supporting compliance with purchasing control requirements under 21 CFR 820.50. Other documents serve different administrative or process functions. SubChapter: Supplier Quality.

Q315. Answer: B

Explanation: Part 806 specifies when manufacturers must report corrections or removals to mitigate health risks or violations. It ensures transparent communication with FDA during recalls or field actions. SubChapter: FDA CFR – Corrections.

Q316. Answer: A

Explanation: Clause 8.2.4 mandates internal audits to confirm QMS conformance to planned arrangements and standards. Audit results drive corrective and preventive actions, ensuring continuous improvement of quality performance. SubChapter: ISO 13485 – Auditing.

Q317. Answer: A

Explanation: Section 820.20 assigns top management responsibility for QMS establishment, implementation, and maintenance. Leadership must ensure adequate resources and conduct management reviews for effectiveness. SubChapter: QSR – Management Responsibility.

Q318. Answer: A

Explanation: Article 83 mandates manufacturers to establish and maintain a PMS system to collect and analyze post-market data. It supports vigilance and corrective actions to ensure ongoing compliance and safety. SubChapter: EU MDR – PMS.

Q319. Answer: D

Explanation: Clause 7.3 defines design and development requirements, including planning, input/output, review, verification, and validation stages. It ensures systematic and documented product realization. SubChapter: ISO 13485 – Design.

Q320. Answer: A

Explanation: Section 704 grants FDA authority to inspect any facility involved in medical device manufacture or holding to assess regulatory compliance. It is the legal foundation for routine and for-cause inspections. SubChapter: FD&C Act – Inspection.

Q321. Answer: A

Explanation: Section 820.72 mandates calibration and maintenance of inspection and test equipment to ensure measurement accuracy. Missing calibration records indicate nonconformance under equipment control requirements. SubChapter: QSR – Equipment Control.

Q322. Answer: A

Explanation: Part 11 requires secure user authentication, audit trails, and integrity safeguards for electronic records and signatures. It ensures data authenticity and traceability equivalent to paper-based records. SubChapter: FDA CFR – Electronic Records.

Q323. Answer: B

Explanation: Inadequate sterilization validation violates 21 CFR 820.75, which mandates validation of processes whose results cannot be fully verified. This ensures consistent product safety and sterility assurance. SubChapter: QSR – Validation.

Q324. Answer: A

Explanation: Clause 7.2.3 covers customer communication regarding product information, feedback, and complaints. Effective interaction ensures issues are addressed promptly and compliance is maintained. SubChapter: ISO 13485 – Communication.

Q325. Answer: C

Explanation: CAPA logs must demonstrate investigation, root cause analysis, corrective action, and effectiveness verification. It proves the manufacturer systematically prevents issue recurrence. SubChapter: QSR – CAPA.

Q326. Answer: A

Explanation: Clause 5.5.2 requires a management representative responsible for ensuring QMS conformity and promoting awareness of regulatory requirements within the organization. SubChapter: ISO 13485 – Management.

Q327. Answer: A

Explanation: Article 83 requires updating and improving the PMS plan when data reveal increased risks or trends. Continuous monitoring ensures ongoing safety and compliance. SubChapter: EU MDR – PMS.

Q328. Answer: D

Explanation: Section 304 authorizes FDA to seize devices violating the Act, including adulterated or misbranded products. It supports enforcement and public protection. SubChapter: FD&C Act – Enforcement.

Q329. Answer: A

Explanation: Clause 7.3.8 mandates design transfer to verify production specifications match design outputs, ensuring devices are manufactured consistently and safely. SubChapter: ISO 13485 – Design Transfer.

Q330. Answer: A

Explanation: Section 820.30(f) requires documented verification confirming design outputs meet input requirements. Lack of evidence demonstrates poor design control compliance. SubChapter: QSR – Design Verification.

Q331. Answer: B

Explanation: Vigilance reporting communicates serious incidents and corrective actions to authorities, minimizing risks and ensuring transparency across markets. SubChapter: EU MDR – Vigilance.

Q332. Answer: A

Explanation: Clause 8.5.2 mandates corrective actions to address root causes of detected nonconformities and verify their effectiveness. This supports continual improvement and compliance. SubChapter: ISO 13485 – Corrective Action.

Q333. Answer: A

Explanation: Clause 7.3.9 requires design changes to be identified, reviewed, verified, validated, and approved before implementation. Undocumented changes pose major compliance risks. SubChapter: ISO 13485 – Design Change.

Q334. Answer: A

Explanation: Section 820.198 requires manufacturers to establish complaint handling procedures, including evaluation, investigation, and response documentation. Complaints must be analyzed for CAPA relevance. SubChapter: QSR – Complaints.

Q335. Answer: A

Explanation: Clause 4.1 requires organizations to control outsourced processes that affect product conformity, maintaining responsibility for compliance even when activities are subcontracted. SubChapter: ISO 13485 – Outsourcing.

Q336. Answer: D

Explanation: Manufacturers must evaluate the change under supplier control procedures to determine whether revalidation or notification is required. Risk-based assessment ensures continued compliance. SubChapter: Supplier Management.

Q337. Answer: B

Explanation: Clause 8.4 mandates analysis of feedback, including complaints, audit data, and service reports, to identify improvement opportunities and prevent recurrence. SubChapter: ISO 13485 – Feedback Evaluation.

Q338. Answer: B

Explanation: Part 821 requires manufacturers to track specified devices to ensure recall effectiveness and patient safety. It enables rapid retrieval of affected products when issues arise. SubChapter: FDA CFR – Tracking.

Q339. Answer: A

Explanation: The manufacturer must renew its CE marking certification through conformity reassessment by the notified body to maintain market access and compliance under MDR. SubChapter: EU MDR – Certification.

Q340. Answer: A

Explanation: Clause 7.4.3 mandates purchasing information to specify requirements for products, processes, and acceptance criteria to ensure supplier compliance and traceability. SubChapter: ISO 13485 – Purchasing.

Q341. Answer: A

Explanation: Clause 7.5.9 requires traceability to identify product status throughout production and delivery, ensuring defective batches are isolated during recalls or audits. Traceability maintains linkage between raw materials, components, and final devices. SubChapter: ISO 13485 – Traceability.

Q342. Answer: A

Explanation: Part 807 requires device manufacturers, initial importers, and repackagers to register facilities and list products with FDA before marketing, providing oversight and traceability. Other parts address adverse events, corrections, or tracking. SubChapter: FDA CFR – Registration.

Q343. Answer: B

Explanation: Clause 7.3.9 covers design changes and requires evaluation and verification of updates, including risk analyses. Modifying risk documentation after failures demonstrates responsive design control and continuous improvement. SubChapter: ISO 13485 – Design Change.

Q344. Answer: A

Explanation: Annex III defines requirements for technical documentation and PMS plans, ensuring systematic post-market monitoring and feedback integration into the QMS. Other annexes address conformity, evaluation, and assessment. SubChapter: EU MDR – PMS.

Q345. Answer: A

Explanation: Section 302 empowers federal courts to issue injunctions preventing continued distribution of devices violating the Act. This is one of FDA's key enforcement mechanisms to protect public health. SubChapter: FD&C Act – Enforcement.

Q346. Answer: A

Explanation: Clause 6.2 requires maintaining competence through training, awareness, and evaluation of effectiveness. Failure to train on new SOPs violates this fundamental requirement. SubChapter: ISO 13485 – Competence.

Q347. Answer: D

Explanation: Section 820.40 mandates documents to be reviewed, approved, and dated by authorized personnel before use, preventing errors and ensuring accountability in QMS documentation control. SubChapter: QSR – Document Control.

Q348. Answer: A

Explanation: Clause 8.2.3 requires monitoring and measurement of processes to verify QMS effectiveness and conformity to planned results, forming the basis for corrective actions. SubChapter: ISO 13485 – Process Monitoring.

Q349. Answer: A

Explanation: Management should promptly submit a CAPA plan detailing root cause, corrective actions, and completion dates to address the violation and demonstrate compliance restoration. SubChapter: FDA CFR – Enforcement.

Q350. Answer: A

Explanation: Clause 6.4 mandates control of work environment conditions to prevent contamination and ensure product quality, especially in cleanroom manufacturing or sterilization areas. SubChapter: ISO 13485 – Environment.

Q351. Answer: A

Explanation: Article 10 defines manufacturers' obligations to implement a QMS, maintain technical documentation, and ensure device conformity and vigilance reporting throughout the product lifecycle. SubChapter: EU MDR – Obligations.

Q352. Answer: C

Explanation: The manufacturer must perform supplier re-evaluation and risk assessment per clause 7.4 to confirm continued ability to meet requirements and maintain compliance. SubChapter: Supplier Management.

Q353. Answer: B

Explanation: Part 830 establishes the Unique Device Identification system, requiring standardized codes for traceability and safety monitoring across the device lifecycle. SubChapter: FDA CFR – UDI.

Q354. Answer: A

Explanation: Preventive maintenance records demonstrate compliance with 21 CFR 820.70(g) and ensure equipment reliability through planned servicing, minimizing process variability and device defects. SubChapter: QSR – Maintenance.

Q355. Answer: A

Explanation: Repeated software malfunctions indicate systemic issues requiring CAPA initiation per §820.100. Corrective actions ensure root causes are addressed and recurrence prevented. SubChapter: QSR – Complaint Handling.

Q356. Answer: A

Explanation: Clause 7.3.5 mandates documented design reviews at planned stages to evaluate adequacy, detect problems, and ensure alignment with requirements. SubChapter: ISO 13485 – Design Review.

Q357. Answer: A

Explanation: Section 515 authorizes FDA to require Premarket Approval (PMA) for Class III devices to ensure safety and effectiveness before marketing. SubChapter: FD&C Act – Premarket Approval.

Q358. Answer: D

Explanation: Manufacturers must immediately notify competent authorities and initiate risk assessment and corrective actions under vigilance and PMS provisions to prevent harm. SubChapter: EU MDR – Vigilance.

Q359. Answer: A

Explanation: Clause 8.5.1 requires planned, documented actions to enhance QMS effectiveness, leveraging audit results, data analysis, and corrective efforts to drive continuous improvement. SubChapter: ISO 13485 – Improvement.

Q360. Answer: A
Explanation: Inconsistent sensor readings indicate potential equipment malfunction requiring investigation, calibration verification, and revalidation before continuing production. Ensuring data accuracy maintains process control integrity. SubChapter: QSR – Validation.
Q361. Answer: A
Explanation: Section 820.30(g) mandates design validation using production-equivalent units under defined conditions to confirm the device meets user needs and intended use. Validation includes clinical evaluation when applicable and ensures total design adequacy. SubChapter: QSR – Design Validation.
Q362. Answer: C
Explanation: Clause 4.2.1 requires establishing documented procedures for QMS, including manual, policy, objectives, and interaction of processes. It ensures traceable, consistent implementation across the organization supporting regulatory compliance. SubChapter: ISO 13485 – Documentation.
Q363. Answer: A
Explanation: CAPA effectiveness must be reviewed to confirm corrective actions eliminated the root cause. Without verification, recurrence risk remains high, violating §820.100 requirements for maintaining evidence of successful remediation. SubChapter: QSR – CAPA Effectiveness.
Q364. Answer: A
Explanation: Clause 5.3 requires top management to establish a documented quality policy that supports strategic direction, continuous improvement, and regulatory compliance, ensuring organizational alignment with customer and statutory needs. SubChapter: ISO 13485 – Leadership.
Q365. Answer: A
Explanation: Article 86 requires periodic safety update reports (PSURs) for Class IIa and above devices, summarizing PMS data and conclusions. Missing updates reflect inadequate post-market surveillance and regulatory oversight. SubChapter: EU MDR – PMS.
Q366. Answer: D
Explanation: Management review and internal audit reports are exempt from direct FDA inspection; however, evidence of implementation may be requested. Other records remain accessible during inspections. SubChapter: FDA CFR – Records.
Q367. Answer: A
Explanation: Process revalidation is required whenever manufacturing changes could impact sterilization effectiveness or product specifications. 21 CFR 820.75 demands proof of continued process control. SubChapter: QSR – Validation.
Q368. Answer: A
Explanation: Section 516 permits FDA to ban devices posing unreasonable and substantial risk to health, even when used as intended. This protective measure supplements recall and remedy authorities under other sections. SubChapter: FD&C Act – Safety Enforcement.
Q369. Answer: A
Explanation: Clause 7.5.3.2 demands clear identification of product status throughout production and storage to prevent mix-ups and non-released product distribution, ensuring traceability and control. SubChapter: ISO 13485 – Production Control.
Q370. Answer: D
Explanation: Failure to verify CAPA effectiveness violates §820.100(a)(4), as root-cause actions must be checked for sustained resolution. Repeat occurrences show ineffective problem closure and require management re-evaluation. SubChapter: QSR – CAPA Verification.
Q371. Answer: A
Explanation: Annex IX defines QMS requirements for conformity assessment under MDR 2017/745, including design documentation and production controls audited by notified bodies for CE certification. SubChapter: EU MDR – QMS Assessment.

Q372. Answer: A
Explanation: Section 820.22 requires planned periodic internal audits to verify QMS conformity and effectiveness, with management review of results and timely corrections. Unscheduled checks may complement but not replace this requirement. SubChapter: QSR – Auditing.
Q373. Answer: A
Explanation: Clause 7.4.1 demands evaluation and re-evaluation of suppliers based on their ability to meet specified requirements. Persistent failures trigger review and potential disqualification to maintain QMS integrity. SubChapter: ISO 13485 – Purchasing.
Q374. Answer: D
Explanation: 21 CFR 807 Subpart B covers foreign manufacturer registration and U.S. agent designation, ensuring FDA communication for imported medical devices. SubChapter: FDA CFR – Registration.
Q375. Answer: A
Explanation: Section 820.70(i) requires validation of software used in production or testing to ensure intended performance. Using unvalidated software compromises data integrity and compliance. SubChapter: QSR – Software Validation.
Q376. Answer: A
Explanation: Clause 7.1 requires risk management integration across product realization, ensuring identified hazards are controlled and monitored during design and manufacture. SubChapter: ISO 13485 – Risk Management.
Q377. Answer: A
Explanation: Section 820.120 covers labeling controls, requiring inspection and storage procedures to prevent mix-ups. Failure to segregate or verify labels can lead to serious safety issues. SubChapter: QSR – Labeling Control.
Q378. Answer: D
Explanation: Section 704 allows FDA to inspect records and facilities to determine compliance with the Act and QSR requirements. This authority supports routine and for-cause inspections. SubChapter: FD&C Act – Inspection Authority.
Q379. Answer: A
Explanation: Clause 7.3.2 requires identification and recording of design inputs to ensure product requirements are complete and verifiable before development. Missing inputs create design gaps and nonconformance risks. SubChapter: ISO 13485 – Design Input.
Q380. Answer: A
Explanation: Section 820.25 requires manufacturers to document employee training and verify its effectiveness to ensure qualified personnel perform regulated tasks correctly. Training records must be maintained and reviewed during inspections. SubChapter: QSR – Training.
Q381. Answer: A
Explanation: 21 CFR Part 11 governs electronic records and electronic signatures, ensuring authenticity, integrity, and confidentiality of digital documentation. It establishes equivalence with traditional paper-based signatures for regulatory compliance. SubChapter: FDA CFR – Electronic Systems.
Q382. Answer: A
Explanation: Clause 7.1 requires applying risk management during product realization, particularly for software and AI components, ensuring continuous assessment of algorithm reliability and patient safety impacts. SubChapter: ISO 13485 – Risk Integration.
Q383. Answer: C
Explanation: Article 13 outlines importer responsibilities to verify CE marking, documentation, and device registration before placing products on the EU market. It ensures supply chain accountability and traceability. SubChapter: EU MDR – Importer Duties.
Q384. Answer: A

Explanation: Electronic complaint systems must maintain data integrity, security, and complete audit trails per 21 CFR 820.198 and Part 11. These safeguards prevent unauthorized edits and support regulatory traceability. SubChapter: QSR – Complaint Handling.

Q385. Answer: A

Explanation: Blockchain provides transparency, but manufacturers remain responsible for validating electronic data integrity and verifying supplier compliance under §820.50 and ISO 13485:7.4. SubChapter: Supplier Quality – Digital Integration.

Q386. Answer: A

Explanation: Section 522 authorizes FDA to require postmarket surveillance for certain Class II and III devices to monitor long-term safety and performance through active data collection. SubChapter: FD&C Act – Postmarket Studies.

Q387. Answer: D

Explanation: Auditors review electronic audit trails recording user actions, timestamps, and data changes to confirm integrity, completeness, and accountability within the QMS. SubChapter: QSR – Data Integrity.

Q388. Answer: A

Explanation: Calibration records must document equipment identification, results, and acceptance criteria to prove measurement accuracy and traceability to standards, ensuring reliable product conformity verification. SubChapter: ISO 13485 – Calibration.

Q389. Answer: A

Explanation: Annex II defines the structure of technical documentation, including device description, design, risk management, and verification/validation data necessary for conformity assessment. SubChapter: EU MDR – Technical Documentation.

Q390. Answer: A

Explanation: Software modifications altering intended use or performance require design change review and potential revalidation under §820.30(i) and ISO 13485:7.3.9 to ensure maintained safety and efficacy. SubChapter: Software Lifecycle – Design Control.

Q391. Answer: D

Explanation: Clause 7.5.7 mandates validating sterilization processes and maintaining controlled conditions to ensure sterility assurance. Deviations require requalification before production continuation. SubChapter: ISO 13485 – Sterilization.

Q392. Answer: A

Explanation: Manufacturers must submit Medical Device Reports (MDRs) electronically via the FDA eMDR gateway to streamline analysis and ensure prompt event tracking. SubChapter: FDA CFR – MDR Reporting.

Q393. Answer: A

Explanation: Clause 8.4 requires analyzing quality data, including feedback, complaints, and statistical trends, to identify nonconformities and drive continuous improvement—modern analytics enhance this process. SubChapter: ISO 13485 – Data Analysis.

Q394. Answer: A

Explanation: Section 305 provides for notice of opportunity for hearing before legal enforcement actions, effectively the warning letter phase signaling corrective action necessity. SubChapter: FD&C Act – Compliance Notice.

Q395. Answer: D

Explanation: FDA and notified bodies must have access to electronic QMS data regardless of hosting location to verify compliance. Transparency and traceability remain manufacturer responsibilities. SubChapter: QMS Infrastructure – Digital Compliance.

Q396. Answer: A

Explanation: Clause 8.5.2 requires verifying corrective action effectiveness before closure to ensure root causes are eliminated and issues do not recur, maintaining process reliability and safety. SubChapter: ISO 13485 – CAPA.

Q397. Answer: A

Explanation: Article 33 establishes EUDAMED, the European database providing public and regulatory access to device information, vigilance data, and certificates, enhancing transparency across the EU market. SubChapter: EU MDR – Transparency.

Q398. Answer: A

Explanation: Device History Record (DHR) and Unique Device Identification (UDI) systems provide traceable production and distribution information enabling rapid recall or investigation response to regulatory requests. SubChapter: QSR – Traceability.

Q399. Answer: C

Explanation: Clause 8.2.1 requires collecting and analyzing feedback to improve product safety and reduce risks through proactive identification of systemic weaknesses. SubChapter: ISO 13485 – Feedback.

Q400. Answer: A

Explanation: EU IVDR Article 56 mandates continuous performance evaluation and PMS for IVDs using real-time data to demonstrate analytical and clinical reliability throughout their lifecycle. SubChapter: EU IVDR – PMS.

Questions (401-500)

Q401. Under ISO 13485, clause 4.2.4 requires records to be:

A. Legible, retrievable, identifiable

B. Encrypted, hidden, confidential

C. Optional, temporary, brief

D. Manual, unverified, flexible

Q402. Scenario: A new sterilization contractor is hired. What must the manufacturer perform first?

A. Supplier qualification audit

B. Cost evaluation

C. Label inspection

D. Marketing review

Q403. 21 CFR 820.181 requires the Device Master Record to include:

A. Price lists

B. Financial reports

C. Marketing materials

D. Manufacturing instructions

Q404. Scenario: A design team introduces a new biocompatible polymer. What must be done first?

A. Design verification

B. Marketing approval

C. Shelf labeling

D. Distributor training

Q405. Which FD&C Act section allows FDA to detain imported medical devices?

A. 801(a)

B. 515

C. 518

D. 704

Q406. Under ISO 13485 clause 8.2.2, customer feedback must be used to:

A. Improve product safety and performance

B. Approve marketing campaigns

C. Set executive bonuses

D. Estimate delivery cost

Q407. Scenario: An FDA inspector notes missing CAPA trend charts. Which process is deficient?

A. CAPA effectiveness monitoring

B. Label printing control

C. Resource planning

D. Software validation

Q408. What is the objective of ISO 13485 clause 8.3 on nonconforming product?

A. Reduce supplier count

B. Simplify labeling processes

C. Prevent unintended use or delivery

D. Lower audit frequency

Q409. Scenario: During EU MDR surveillance, the notified body requests PSUR analysis. What is expected?

A. PMS trend evaluation

B. Financial summary

C. Supplier list

D. HR training records

Q410. Which FDA CFR section covers labeling control for medical devices?
A. 820.120
B. 820.70
C. 820.50
D. 820.180
Q411. Scenario: Cloud QMS users modify audit records post-approval. Which regulation is breached?
A. 21 CFR Part 11
B. 21 CFR 807
C. 21 CFR 830
D. 21 CFR 801
Q412. ISO 13485 clause 6.3 mandates management of:
A. Financial assets
B. Marketing teams
C. Infrastructure and facilities
D. Sales strategies
Q413. Scenario: A supplier introduces automated inspection. What must the manufacturer verify?
A. Equipment validation results
B. Supplier branding
C. Worker uniforms
D. Invoice approvals
Q414. Which FD&C Act section authorizes voluntary recalls?
A. 518(e)
B. 510(a)
C. 516(b)
D. 704(d)
Q415. Scenario: An EU manufacturer upgrades cybersecurity features in connected devices. What must be updated?
A. Risk management file
B. CE logo
C. Shelf labeling
D. Pricing chart
Q416. Under ISO 13485 clause 5.6, management reviews must include:
A. Competitor data, trade shows, media reach
B. Marketing metrics, sales revenue, inventory
C. Audit results, feedback, process performance
D. Employee schedules, leave requests, costs
Q417. Scenario: A complaint reveals device malfunction caused by supplier subcomponent. What must be initiated?
A. Supplier CAPA
B. Product redesign
C. HR review
D. Distributor survey
Q418. What is the purpose of FDA's Quality System Inspection Technique (QSIT)?
A. Standardize inspection focus
B. Replace audits
C. Control budgets
D. Approve new devices

Q419. Scenario: Data from a PMS system indicate increased adverse events in a specific region. What must the manufacturer do?
A. Conduct trend analysis and notify regulators
B. Pause marketing
C. Change product name
D. Modify packaging
Q420. According to ISO 13485, clause 7.3.3 requires design outputs to:
A. Follow marketing plan
B. Be visually attractive
C. Reduce costs
D. Meet input requirements
Q421. Under 21 CFR 820.75, process validation must include:
A. Defined acceptance criteria
B. Verbal approval only
C. Temporary records
D. Supplier consent
Q422. Scenario: An auditor reviews a manufacturer's training files and finds missing evaluation of training effectiveness. Which clause applies?
A. ISO 13485:6.2
B. ISO 13485:5.6
C. ISO 13485:7.4
D. ISO 13485:8.3
Q423. According to EU MDR, Article 87 requires manufacturers to report serious incidents:
A. Without delay
B. Annually only
C. After product recall
D. At supplier's request
Q424. Scenario: A supplier implements a new automated welding process. What must the manufacturer verify first?
A. Packaging changes
B. Supplier turnover data
C. Process validation evidence
D. Audit frequency
Q425. Which FD&C Act section authorizes FDA to require registration and listing of device manufacturers?
A. Section 510
B. Section 301
C. Section 704
D. Section 518
Q426. Scenario: During inspection, an FDA investigator requests design review meeting records. Which regulation applies?
A. 21 CFR 820.30(e)
B. 21 CFR 820.90
C. 21 CFR 820.180
D. 21 CFR 820.50
Q427. ISO 13485 clause 7.5.8 requires product cleanliness to be maintained:
A. During production and packaging
B. Before financial closure

C. Only after shipping
D. Before auditing
Q428. Scenario: A complaint reveals recurring battery overheating. What is the manufacturer's first regulatory obligation?
A. Contact distributors
B. Conduct market survey
C. Evaluate for MDR reporting
D. Revise labels immediately
Q429. What is the objective of ISO 13485 clause 4.1 regarding process outsourcing?
A. Maintain control and accountability
B. Transfer full responsibility
C. Reduce audit obligations
D. Delegate certification
Q430. Scenario: A cybersecurity breach exposes connected device data. Under EU MDR Annex I, what must be demonstrated?
A. Data protection and system resilience
B. Supplier consent
C. Financial loss estimation
D. Label color matching
Q431. Under 21 CFR 820.100, effectiveness checks for corrective actions must be:
A. Documented and verified
B. Verbal and optional
C. Informal and temporary
D. Cost-driven only
Q432. Scenario: An IVD manufacturer adds real-time patient monitoring functions. What must be updated in technical documentation?
A. Distributor contracts
B. Warranty period only
C. Sales projections
D. Risk management and performance evaluation
Q433. Which FD&C Act section permits mandatory recalls for imminent hazards?
A. 518(e)
B. 515(b)
C. 704(a)
D. 522(c)
Q434. Scenario: A device label translation error is discovered in the EU. What must the manufacturer initiate?
A. Field Safety Corrective Action
B. Product redesign
C. Supplier audit
D. Contract termination
Q435. ISO 13485 clause 8.2.4 requires internal audit programs to:
A. Verify QMS conformity and effectiveness
B. Replace management review
C. Focus only on finance
D. Occur after product recall
Q436. Scenario: FDA requests a 48-hour turnaround on CAPA summaries. Which documentation should be provided?

A. Supplier invoice folder
B. Marketing expense sheet
C. Equipment maintenance log
D. CAPA master log with status, root cause, and verification data

Q437. Which EU MDR article defines requirements for unique device identification assignment?
A. Article 27
B. Article 10
C. Article 33
D. Article 61

Q438. Scenario: A process deviation is found during production but product meets specifications. What should be done?
A. Document and assess deviation under nonconformance procedures
B. Ignore event
C. Approve shipment immediately
D. Re-label product silently

Q439. Which FD&C Act section empowers FDA to inspect facilities for compliance?
A. 704
B. 510
C. 515
D. 518

Q440. Scenario: A cloud-hosted QMS loses connectivity during an audit. What must the organization demonstrate?
A. Design label copy
B. Marketing contingency plan
C. Contract renegotiation
D. Data backup, recovery, and accessibility procedures

Q441. Modern eQMS solutions supporting remote audits must comply with which regulatory expectation?
A. 21 CFR Part 11
B. 21 CFR 820 Subpart M
C. ISO 13485 Clause 6.2
D. EU MDR Annex XI

Q442. Scenario: A manufacturer introduces machine-learning algorithms to optimize device calibration. What must be demonstrated?
A. Software validation and risk control
B. Marketing budget approval
C. Supplier pricing agreement
D. Audit team rotation

Q443. Which ISO 13485 clause requires documented evidence of environmental controls for clean manufacturing areas?
A. 6.4
B. 7.5.9
C. 8.3.2
D. 5.5.1

Q444. Scenario: A CAPA trend report shows rising software defects post-update. What should management do first?
A. Pause training sessions
B. Notify media

C. Initiate root cause investigation
D. Request budget increase
Q445. EU MDR Article 61 requires clinical evaluation to demonstrate:
A. Safety and performance based on clinical evidence
B. Marketing success potential
C. Production efficiency
D. Labeling consistency
Q446. Scenario: A supplier transitions to 3D-printed components. What must the manufacturer obtain before approval?
A. Process validation and material certification records
B. Cost comparison table
C. Employee shift schedule
D. Marketing presentation
Q447. Under ISO 13485 clause 7.3.7, design transfer activities must ensure:
A. Manufacturing outputs match approved design specifications
B. Promotional materials are updated
C. Auditors are replaced annually
D. Finance records are aligned
Q448. Scenario: Cloud-based device testing data is stored in multiple regions. What must the manufacturer guarantee?
A. Data integrity and regulatory access to records
B. Supplier exclusivity
C. Marketing permissions
D. Time-zone alignment
Q449. According to ISO 13485 clause 8.5.3, preventive actions must:
A. Be handled by finance department
B. Be taken after market withdrawal only
C. Replace complaint investigations
D. Address potential nonconformities before occurrence
Q450. Scenario: A manufacturer uses a digital dashboard for real-time CAPA metrics. What benefit must be demonstrated to auditors?
A. Objective evidence of data accuracy and timely follow-up
B. Marketing engagement
C. Supplier reduction
D. Price optimization
Q451. FDA 21 CFR 820.198 requires complaints to be:
A. Evaluated and investigated for reportability
B. Filed only after recall
C. Handled by sales teams
D. Deleted after review
Q452. Scenario: An EU manufacturer integrates AI diagnostics into an existing Class IIb device. What must be updated first?
A. Clinical evaluation and risk file
B. Distribution contracts
C. Marketing strategy
D. Shipping routes
Q453. ISO 13485 clause 8.4 requires data analysis to include:
A. Sales forecasts

B. Advertising reach
C. Complaints, process trends, and supplier performance
D. Inventory aging

Q454. Scenario: An auditor requests evidence of device traceability post-distribution. Which system must the firm reference?
A. UDI and DHR records
B. Marketing archives
C. Payroll software
D. Vendor quotations

Q455. FD&C Act Section 516 empowers FDA to:
A. Ban devices posing substantial risk
B. Fund product development
C. Set international pricing
D. Market new technologies

Q456. Scenario: During validation, sensor data fluctuates beyond tolerance. What must be done immediately?
A. Investigate root cause and revalidate process
B. Ignore variation
C. Ship product quickly
D. Delete results

Q457. ISO 13485 clause 7.5.6 requires software used in production to be:
A. Costed in budgets
B. Reviewed monthly by HR
C. Validated for intended purpose before use
D. Removed after testing

Q458. Scenario: Post-market trend data show higher failure rates in one region. What action is required?
A. Perform root cause analysis and submit report to authorities
B. Change product name
C. Switch marketing agency
D. Reduce pricing

Q459. Under 21 CFR 820.180, records must be:
A. Readable, readily available, and maintained for device lifecycle
B. Destroyed after five days
C. Stored only on paper
D. Archived without indexing

Q460. Scenario: An EU MDR audit requests evidence of post-market performance follow-up (PMPF). What document must be submitted?
A. Updated PMS Plan and PMPF Report
B. Sales brochure
C. Supplier invoice
D. Product catalog

Q461. A manufacturer identifies microbial contamination in a cleanroom. Which ISO standard primarily governs airborne particulate control for medical device environments?
A. ISO 13485
B. ISO 14971
C. ISO 14644
D. ISO 11135

Q462. During a risk analysis session, the team identifies a potential device failure causing minor user injury. According to ISO 14971, what is the next step?
A. Accept the risk as negligible
B. Implement risk control measures
C. Document and ignore the event
D. Wait for regulatory inspection
Q463. Which FDA regulation governs medical device labeling requirements, including intended use and warnings?
A. 21 CFR 820
B. 21 CFR 803
C. 21 CFR 801
D. 21 CFR 11
Q464. A firm designing an infusion pump must validate embedded software. Which international standard specifies the lifecycle framework for this validation?
A. ISO 13485
B. IEC 62304
C. ISO 9001
D. ISO 17025
Q465. A packaging engineer evaluates shelf-life and seal integrity for a sterile catheter. Which ISO series is most relevant?
A. ISO 11135
B. ISO 11607
C. ISO 13485
D. ISO 14644
Q466. A device reprocessing facility must ensure sterilization validation aligns with which ISO standard for ethylene oxide processes?
A. ISO 11137
B. ISO 11135
C. ISO 14644
D. ISO 13485
Q467. A new blood glucose meter undergoes usability testing revealing frequent user errors. Under FDA design control (21 CFR 820.30), what must the manufacturer do next?
A. Update labeling only
B. Submit a PMA supplement immediately
C. Discontinue the product
D. Perform corrective design review
Q468. Which process best ensures consistent sterile barrier performance across production batches?
A. Sampling during final inspection only
B. Sterilization load mapping and process validation
C. End-user feedback tracking
D. Increasing EtO concentration randomly
Q469. Which clause of ISO 13485 directly addresses design and development validation?
A. 7.3.7
B. 8.5.2
C. 6.2
D. 4.2.3
Q470. A product team evaluates biological safety of materials contacting blood. Which ISO standard applies?

A. ISO 10993
B. ISO 11607
C. ISO 11137
D. ISO 13485

Q471. A sterilization engineer monitors dose audits for gamma-irradiated products. Which ISO document governs this?
A. ISO 11137
B. ISO 11135
C. ISO 14644
D. ISO 13485

Q472. The UDI (Unique Device Identification) requirement improves:
A. Sales forecasting
B. Supply chain traceability
C. Material recycling
D. Marketing strategies

Q473. Which document should a design team reference to integrate usability engineering principles?
A. IEC 62366
B. ISO 11137
C. ISO 14644
D. ISO 9001

Q474. A CAPA team identifies process contamination due to inadequate HEPA maintenance. What validation step ensures correction effectiveness?
A. Cleaning frequency reduction
B. HEPA integrity test per ISO 14644-3
C. Packaging redesign
D. Label change

Q475. Which global regulation focuses on post-market surveillance and vigilance for medical devices?
A. ISO 13485 Clause 8
B. EU MDR 2017/745 Chapter VII
C. 21 CFR 820 Subpart C
D. ISO 9001 Clause 10

Q476. In failure analysis, which method identifies crack initiation sites in metal implants?
A. FTIR Spectroscopy
B. Scanning Electron Microscopy (SEM)
C. X-Ray Fluorescence (XRF)
D. High-Performance Liquid Chromatography (HPLC)

Q477. A manufacturer validates cleaning effectiveness before sterilization. Which measurement ensures no residual protein remains?
A. TOC Analysis
B. Bioburden Count
C. Endotoxin Test
D. Visual Inspection

Q478. Which international standard defines risk management for medical device software?
A. IEC 62304 Annex C
B. ISO 14971 Annex E
C. ISO 13485 Clause 7.1
D. ISO 14644 Part 2

Q479. What test ensures sterilant penetration during EtO cycle development?

A. Half-cycle biological indicator testing
B. Endotoxin test
C. Colorimetric label check
D. Residual gas analysis only

Q480. Which analytical tool supports design verification by linking user needs to engineering specifications?
A. Ishikawa diagram
B. Design Failure Mode and Effects Analysis (DFMEA)
C. House of Quality (QFD)
D. Fishbone diagram

Q481. During validation of a new cleanroom, temperature and humidity were within range but airborne particulates exceeded ISO Class 7 limits. What action should be taken?
A. Continue production under deviation
B. Perform root-cause investigation and requalify
C. Replace filters without testing
D. Accept temporary non-conformance

Q482. A design engineer revises labeling to add a new storage condition. Which document must be updated first?
A. Device master record (DMR)
B. Device history record (DHR)
C. Management review minutes
D. Supplier evaluation file

Q483. A device uses sterilization by moist heat. Which validation step confirms uniform steam penetration?
A. Thermometric distribution study
B. Half-cycle biological test
C. Bioburden enumeration
D. Chemical-indicator color check

Q484. Risk analysis identifies electrical shock potential from insulation degradation. What is the best mitigation?
A. Add software lockouts
B. Strengthen insulation material and retest
C. Increase labeling warnings
D. Reduce inspection frequency

Q485. Which FDA requirement enforces verification that design outputs meet input requirements?
A. 21 CFR 820.30(f)
B. 21 CFR 820.70
C. 21 CFR 820.198
D. 21 CFR 820.90

Q486. A developer applies IEC 62304 Class C to life-support software. What does this classification signify?
A. Failure causes no injury
B. Failure could cause minor injury
C. Failure could lead to death or serious injury
D. Software not regulated

Q487. Which sterilization documentation element provides evidence of ongoing process control?
A. Validation protocol
B. Routine monitoring records

C. Installation qualification
D. Supplier audit report

Q488. A design review identifies insufficient hazard labeling on a reusable surgical instrument. Which regulation mandates correction?
A. ISO 13485 § 7.3.9
B. 21 CFR 801
C. ISO 9001 § 8.5
D. 21 CFR 820.184

Q489. During packaging validation, burst testing revealed marginal seal strength. What must the engineer do?
A. Adjust sealing parameters and re-validate
B. Continue using current settings
C. Reject only failed samples
D. Add warning labels

Q490. Which standard provides guidance on applying risk management to usability?
A. ISO 14971 Annex C
B. IEC 62366-1
C. ISO 9001 Clause 10
D. IEC 60601-1

Q491. A complaint investigation finds sterilization records missing for a lot. What QSR requirement is violated?
A. Device master record maintenance
B. Process validation documentation
C. Record retention and traceability
D. Design input review

Q492. Which technique determines endotoxin presence after cleaning validation?
A. LAL test
B. TOC analysis
C. Bioburden count
D. UV spectroscopy

Q493. A global manufacturer aligns with both U.S. FDA QSR and EU MDR. Which principle ensures consistency across regions?
A. Process harmonization using ISO 13485
B. Dual documentation for each region
C. Separate QMS for each plant
D. Outsourced compliance responsibility

Q494. A device design includes a lithium battery; risk analysis identifies overheating potential. Which standard provides testing criteria?
A. IEC 62133
B. ISO 14971
C. ISO 13485
D. ISO 11135

Q495. Which type of validation ensures a manufacturing process consistently produces sterile output within specified limits?
A. Installation Qualification
B. Performance Qualification
C. Design Qualification
D. Supplier Qualification

Q496. In design verification, which statistical tool best determines if process variation meets tolerance?

A. Control Chart
B. Regression Analysis
C. Capability Index (Cpk)
D. Pareto Chart

Q497. What activity confirms that risk-control measures implemented are effective and do not introduce new risks?

A. Risk Analysis
B. Risk Evaluation
C. Risk Control Verification
D. Design Validation

Q498. During usability validation, operators repeatedly confuse start and stop buttons. What corrective action aligns with IEC 62366-1?

A. Provide additional training only
B. Redesign interface layout and retest
C. Increase warning text size
D. Add password lockout

Q499. Which cleanroom test verifies pressure differentials between rooms?

A. Airflow Visualization
B. Differential Pressure Mapping
C. Particle Counting
D. HEPA Leak Testing

Q500. A process engineer establishes sterilization cycle alarms for load temperature deviations. What quality principle does this represent?

A. Preventive control
B. Corrective action
C. Process revalidation
D. Supplier qualification

Answer key and Explanation (401-500)

Q401. Answer: A
Explanation: Clause 4.2.4 requires records to be legible, readily identifiable, and retrievable to demonstrate QMS effectiveness and regulatory conformity. Proper documentation supports audits, traceability, and product verification integrity. SubChapter: ISO 13485 – Record Control.
Q402. Answer: A
Explanation: Outsourced sterilization impacts product conformity, requiring supplier qualification and validation audits per ISO 13485:7.4 and 21 CFR 820.50 to ensure process control and compliance. SubChapter: Supplier Quality – Qualification.
Q403. Answer: D
Explanation: The DMR must include manufacturing instructions, specifications, and quality procedures to ensure consistent, controlled production meeting design and regulatory standards. SubChapter: QSR – Documentation.
Q404. Answer: A
Explanation: Any new material introduction requires design verification testing to confirm the change maintains safety, functionality, and compliance with ISO 10993 and §820.30(f) requirements. SubChapter: Design Control – Verification.
Q405. Answer: A
Explanation: Section 801(a) authorizes FDA to detain or refuse entry of imported devices appearing adulterated, misbranded, or noncompliant with the FD&C Act. SubChapter: FD&C Act – Imports.
Q406. Answer: A
Explanation: Clause 8.2.2 requires organizations to analyze customer feedback to improve device safety, reliability, and QMS performance. It's essential for preventive and corrective action planning. SubChapter: ISO 13485 – Feedback.
Q407. Answer: A
Explanation: CAPA systems must include data trend analysis to identify recurring issues and evaluate correction effectiveness under §820.100(a)(1). Missing trend charts signal weak preventive systems. SubChapter: QSR – CAPA Monitoring.
Q408. Answer: C
Explanation: Clause 8.3 ensures that nonconforming product is identified, controlled, and prevented from unintended use or delivery, protecting patient safety and maintaining regulatory compliance. SubChapter: ISO 13485 – Nonconformance.
Q409. Answer: A
Explanation: The PSUR provides analysis of post-market surveillance data, identifying trends, and verifying the continued benefit-risk balance of devices as required under Article 86. SubChapter: EU MDR – PMS.
Q410. Answer: A
Explanation: Section 820.120 requires control over labeling operations, storage, and inspection to prevent mix-ups and ensure labels are accurate and applied correctly. SubChapter: QSR – Labeling.
Q411. Answer: A
Explanation: Part 11 prohibits unauthorized alteration of approved records, requiring audit trails and user authentication to preserve data integrity and regulatory confidence. SubChapter: FDA CFR – Electronic Records.
Q412. Answer: C
Explanation: Clause 6.3 ensures organizations maintain and control infrastructure and facilities necessary to achieve product conformity, including buildings, workspace, and supporting utilities. SubChapter: ISO 13485 – Infrastructure.

Q413. Answer: A
Explanation: When suppliers adopt new technology, manufacturers must verify process validation results to confirm inspection accuracy and maintain product conformity per §820.50 and ISO 13485:7.4. SubChapter: Supplier Quality.
Q414. Answer: A
Explanation: Section 518(e) enables FDA to request or oversee voluntary recalls when devices pose health risks, providing structured withdrawal procedures under 21 CFR 7 guidance. SubChapter: FD&C Act – Recalls.
Q415. Answer: A
Explanation: Cybersecurity updates must be documented within the risk management file to reflect mitigated threats, per ISO 14971 and MDR Annex I safety principles. SubChapter: Risk Management – Cybersecurity.
Q416. Answer: C
Explanation: Clause 5.6 requires management review of audit results, feedback, complaints, process data, and improvement opportunities to ensure QMS effectiveness and compliance. SubChapter: ISO 13485 – Management Review.
Q417. Answer: A
Explanation: When supplier material defects lead to product failure, a supplier CAPA must be initiated to correct root causes and prevent recurrence per §820.50 and ISO 13485:7.4. SubChapter: Supplier Quality – CAPA.
Q418. Answer: A
Explanation: QSIT standardizes FDA inspection methodology into four subsystems—Management Controls, CAPA, Design Controls, and Production Controls—to ensure consistent, comprehensive regulatory oversight. SubChapter: FDA Inspection Systems.
Q419. Answer: A
Explanation: PMS data indicating regional trends require investigation, root-cause analysis, and regulatory notification under MDR Article 83 and ISO 13485:8.4. SubChapter: PMS – Trend Analysis.
Q420. Answer: D
Explanation: Clause 7.3.3 ensures design outputs meet input requirements, providing specifications for manufacturing, testing, and acceptance. Documented traceability between inputs and outputs verifies conformity. SubChapter: ISO 13485 – Design Output.
Q421. Answer: A
Explanation: Section 820.75 requires process validation with documented procedures, predetermined acceptance criteria, and objective evidence that processes consistently produce conforming devices. This ensures ongoing control of critical parameters when inspection alone cannot verify quality, forming a cornerstone of device manufacturing compliance and patient safety. SubChapter: QSR – Validation.
Q422. Answer: A
Explanation: Clause 6.2 of ISO 13485 requires organizations not only to provide training but also to evaluate its effectiveness. Demonstrating competence for personnel performing tasks affecting product quality helps maintain consistent compliance and process control across all regulated manufacturing environments. SubChapter: ISO 13485 – Competence and Training.
Q423. Answer: A
Explanation: Article 87 of EU MDR 2017/745 mandates that manufacturers report serious incidents and field safety corrective actions immediately upon awareness to ensure rapid mitigation. Timely reporting enhances transparency and patient protection under post-market surveillance obligations. SubChapter: EU MDR – Vigilance.
Q424. Answer: C

Explanation: The manufacturer must confirm the supplier's automated welding process has been validated according to ISO 13485:7.4 and 21 CFR 820.75. This ensures the process consistently produces outputs meeting specifications and prevents latent defects in critical assemblies or sterile barriers. SubChapter: Supplier Quality – Validation.

Q425. Answer: A

Explanation: Section 510 mandates registration of device establishments and listing of marketed products. These requirements allow FDA to identify responsible parties, prioritize inspections, and monitor post-market compliance activities, ensuring transparency and traceability within the medical device supply chain. SubChapter: FD&C Act – Registration.

Q426. Answer: A

Explanation: Section 820.30(e) requires formal, documented design reviews at defined stages to assess design adequacy and identify problems before transfer. Records must include participants, conclusions, and any resulting actions. Their absence indicates weak design control and incomplete traceability. SubChapter: QSR – Design Control.

Q427. Answer: A

Explanation: Clause 7.5.8 mandates procedures to maintain product cleanliness during manufacturing, handling, and packaging when contamination could affect device performance or safety. Environmental controls and validated cleaning processes ensure consistent compliance and patient protection. SubChapter: ISO 13485 – Product Cleanliness.

Q428. Answer: C

Explanation: Complaints suggesting serious injury potential require MDR evaluation under 21 CFR 803. Investigation must determine if the event meets reporting criteria and trigger CAPA if systemic root causes exist. SubChapter: FDA CFR – MDR Evaluation.

Q429. Answer: A

Explanation: Clause 4.1 ensures organizations remain responsible for outsourced processes that affect product conformity. Even when external partners perform tasks, the manufacturer must monitor and control quality outcomes, maintaining ultimate accountability for regulatory compliance. SubChapter: ISO 13485 – Outsourced Processes.

Q430. Answer: A

Explanation: Annex I (Chapter II) requires demonstration of cybersecurity and data protection measures throughout device design and lifecycle. Manufacturers must ensure confidentiality, integrity, and availability of data in connected systems. SubChapter: EU MDR – Cybersecurity.

Q431. Answer: A

Explanation: Section 820.100 requires documented verification that corrective actions prevent recurrence. Effectiveness checks confirm root causes were accurately addressed, ensuring sustained compliance and improved process stability. SubChapter: QSR – CAPA Effectiveness.

Q432. Answer: D

Explanation: The addition of patient monitoring capabilities changes device intended use, requiring updated risk management, performance evaluation, and validation records under IVDR Annex II and ISO 14971. SubChapter: IVDR – Design Updates.

Q433. Answer: A

Explanation: Section 518(e) empowers FDA to mandate recalls when devices pose an unreasonable risk of substantial harm, ensuring swift protection of public health. Voluntary recall options often precede this action. SubChapter: FD&C Act – Mandatory Recall.

Q434. Answer: A

Explanation: Labeling inaccuracies affecting safety trigger a Field Safety Corrective Action (FSCA) per EU MDR Article 89. The manufacturer must notify authorities and issue a Field Safety Notice (FSN) to users. SubChapter: EU MDR – Vigilance.

Q435. Answer: A
Explanation: Clause 8.2.4 ensures planned audits evaluate QMS implementation and effectiveness across processes. Audit results must be documented, reported to management, and followed by corrective actions to strengthen system performance. SubChapter: ISO 13485 – Internal Audit.
Q436. Answer: D
Explanation: The CAPA master log consolidates all ongoing and closed CAPAs, including cause, actions, and verification. Providing it demonstrates proactive compliance with §820.100 and management oversight. SubChapter: QSR – CAPA Records.
Q437. Answer: A
Explanation: Article 27 establishes the Unique Device Identification (UDI) system, enhancing traceability across supply chains and facilitating recalls and adverse event investigations. Each device must bear a unique, standardized identifier. SubChapter: EU MDR – UDI.
Q438. Answer: A
Explanation: Even when specifications are met, unapproved deviations require documentation and risk assessment under §820.90 and ISO 13485:8.3. Recording ensures traceability and regulatory transparency during future audits. SubChapter: QSR – Nonconformance.
Q439. Answer: A
Explanation: Section 704 provides FDA with authority to inspect facilities, equipment, and records involved in device manufacturing, ensuring compliance with CGMP and quality system regulations. SubChapter: FD&C Act – Inspection Authority.
Q440. Answer: D
Explanation: Manufacturers using cloud QMS platforms must demonstrate validated backup and data recovery procedures ensuring uninterrupted record accessibility to auditors, per 21 CFR Part 11 and ISO 13485:4.2.4. SubChapter: QMS Infrastructure – Data Integrity.
Q441. Answer: A
Explanation: Electronic QMS platforms require compliance with 21 CFR Part 11 for electronic records and signatures. They must ensure data integrity, security, traceability, and audit trails equivalent to paper records, allowing regulators to verify authenticity during remote or hybrid audits. SubChapter: FDA CFR – Electronic Compliance.
Q442. Answer: A
Explanation: AI-driven processes must undergo software validation under 21 CFR 820.70(i) and risk evaluation per ISO 14971 to confirm they function as intended without introducing uncontrolled risks to device performance or safety. SubChapter: QSR – Software Validation.
Q443. Answer: A
Explanation: Clause 6.4 mandates establishing and maintaining environmental conditions suitable for product quality. Monitoring humidity, temperature, and particulate levels reduces contamination risks for sterile and implantable devices. SubChapter: ISO 13485 – Work Environment.
Q444. Answer: C
Explanation: An increasing trend signals systemic issues requiring immediate root cause investigation per 21 CFR 820.100 and ISO 13485 8.5.2. Effective CAPA identifies design or validation gaps and verifies long-term correction effectiveness. SubChapter: QSR – CAPA Management.
Q445. Answer: A
Explanation: Article 61 mandates clinical evaluation through data analysis and studies to demonstrate safety and performance for intended use. It ensures clinical benefit is supported by scientific evidence prior to CE marking. SubChapter: EU MDR – Clinical Evaluation.
Q446. Answer: A

Explanation: Manufacturers must review 3D-printing validation data and material certificates to verify mechanical and biocompatibility compliance per ISO 13485 7.4 and 21 CFR 820.75. New manufacturing methods require documented qualification. SubChapter: Supplier Control – Additive Manufacturing.

Q447. Answer: A

Explanation: Clause 7.3.7 requires verifying that design outputs are correctly translated into manufacturing specifications, preventing errors during production startup. It ensures consistency between development intent and shop-floor execution. SubChapter: ISO 13485 – Design Transfer.

Q448. Answer: A

Explanation: Manufacturers using cloud repositories must ensure data integrity, traceability, and audit access for regulators per 21 CFR Part 11 and ISO 13485 4.2.4. Geographic distribution cannot limit regulatory oversight or inspection rights. SubChapter: Digital QMS – Data Governance.

Q449. Answer: D

Explanation: Preventive action requires identifying potential issues through trend analysis and risk evaluation to avoid nonconformance. It supports continuous improvement and risk-based thinking in modern QMS operations. SubChapter: ISO 13485 – Preventive Action.

Q450. Answer: A

Explanation: Electronic CAPA tracking tools must show objective accuracy and timely closure of actions. Auditors look for automated trend alerts and verified effectiveness reviews to confirm system control and regulatory maturity. SubChapter: QSR – Digital CAPA Management.

Q451. Answer: A

Explanation: Section 820.198 requires manufacturers to review, evaluate, and investigate each complaint to determine if it must be reported under 21 CFR 803. Proper handling prevents recurrence and enhances safety oversight. SubChapter: FDA CFR – Complaint Handling.

Q452. Answer: A

Explanation: Introducing AI capabilities changes device performance and intended use. Manufacturers must update clinical evaluation and risk documentation under Articles 61 and 83 of EU MDR to confirm continued safety and effectiveness. SubChapter: EU MDR – AI Integration.

Q453. Answer: C

Explanation: Clause 8.4 mandates comprehensive data analysis covering complaints, process capability, and supplier metrics to identify systemic weaknesses. Insights drive CAPA and preventive actions to enhance QMS effectiveness. SubChapter: ISO 13485 – Data Analysis.

Q454. Answer: A

Explanation: Traceability is verified through Unique Device Identification and Device History Record data. These systems enable quick identification of affected units during recalls and support regulatory investigations. SubChapter: QSR – Traceability.

Q455. Answer: A

Explanation: Section 516 allows FDA to ban devices presenting unreasonable or substantial risk to health even when properly used, ensuring rapid response to emerging hazards and protecting patients from unsafe technologies. SubChapter: FD&C Act – Device Ban.

Q456. Answer: A

Explanation: Out-of-tolerance data indicate loss of process control and require root cause investigation followed by revalidation per 820.75 to restore compliance and ensure reliable device output. SubChapter: QSR – Process Validation.

Q457. Answer: C

Explanation: Clause 7.5.6 ensures any software affecting product quality is validated before use to verify consistent, accurate performance. Validation records demonstrate regulatory control over automation tools and data reliability. SubChapter: ISO 13485 – Software Validation.

Q458. Answer: A

Explanation: Regional trend analysis revealing performance issues triggers PMS investigation and regulatory notification under MDR Articles 83 and 84. Timely analysis and reporting prevent escalating risk to patients. SubChapter: PMS – Trend Management.

Q459. Answer: A

Explanation: Section 820.180 requires maintaining records in a readily accessible, legible manner for the entire device lifecycle or minimum retention period, ensuring traceability and regulatory verification readiness. SubChapter: FDA CFR – Record Retention.

Q460. Answer: A

Explanation: Manufacturers must submit an updated PMS plan and PMPF report demonstrating continuous evaluation of clinical performance per MDR Annex XIV Part B. It verifies ongoing safety and effectiveness in real-world use. SubChapter: EU MDR – PMS and PMPF.

Q461. Answer: C

Explanation: ISO 14644 defines cleanroom classifications and particulate limits essential to maintain sterile production environments. Option A addresses QMS requirements, Option B covers risk management, and Option D focuses on sterilization validation, not environmental monitoring. SubChapter: Controlled Environments and Utilities

Q462. Answer: B

Explanation: ISO 14971 requires implementing control measures to reduce risks to acceptable levels. Option A ignores risk management hierarchy, Option C breaches documentation control, and Option D delays mitigation contrary to proactive risk principles. SubChapter: Risk Management

Q463. Answer: C

Explanation: 21 CFR 801 establishes labeling rules ensuring adequate directions for use and identification. Option A covers QSR, Option B concerns adverse event reporting, and Option D addresses electronic records and signatures. SubChapter: Labeling and UDI

Q464. Answer: B

Explanation: IEC 62304 outlines software lifecycle processes for safety classification, verification, and maintenance. Option A defines system-level QMS, Option C is generic to industries, and Option D applies to testing laboratories, not software design. SubChapter: Software Validation

Q465. Answer: B

Explanation: ISO 11607 governs packaging design, validation, and maintenance for terminally sterilized devices. Option A concerns EtO sterilization, Option C addresses QMS, and Option D focuses on environmental particulates, not packaging performance. SubChapter: Design Controls

Q466. Answer: B

Explanation: ISO 11135 specifies EtO sterilization validation and routine control requirements. Option A applies to radiation methods, Option C covers cleanroom control, and Option D defines QMS frameworks rather than sterilization processes. SubChapter: Sterilization

Q467. Answer: D

Explanation: 21 CFR 820.30 requires design reviews addressing user feedback and human factors. Option A may be inadequate, Option C excessive, and Option B premature without assessing design adequacy. SubChapter: Human Factors and Design Control

Q468. Answer: B

Explanation: Load mapping and process validation verify uniform sterilization, assuring barrier integrity. Option A lacks process validation, Option C is reactive, and Option D risks overexposure and product damage. SubChapter: Sterilization Validation

Q469. Answer: A

Explanation: ISO 13485 § 7.3.7 mandates validation under simulated use to confirm products meet requirements. Option B handles CAPA, Option C covers competence, and Option D relates to documentation control. SubChapter: Design Validation

Q470. Answer: A
Explanation: ISO 10993 details biocompatibility testing for materials contacting human tissue or fluids. Option B pertains to packaging, Option C to radiation sterilization, and Option D to QMS, not biological evaluation. SubChapter: Biocompatibility and Testing
Q471. Answer: A
Explanation: ISO 11137 defines validation and routine control for radiation sterilization, including dose audits. Option B is EtO-specific, Option C cleanroom control, and Option D generic QMS. SubChapter: Sterilization
Q472. Answer: B
Explanation: UDI enhances traceability and post-market surveillance by linking devices to production data. Option A and D are commercial, while C pertains to sustainability unrelated to regulatory identification. SubChapter: Labeling and UDI
Q473. Answer: A
Explanation: IEC 62366 provides framework for human factors and usability risk management. Option B covers radiation, Option C environment, and Option D generic QMS, not human interface design. SubChapter: Human Factors Engineering
Q474. Answer: B
Explanation: ISO 14644-3 mandates HEPA leak testing to validate air cleanliness recovery. Option A weakens control, Option C and D address unrelated quality elements. SubChapter: Controlled Environments
Q475. Answer: B
Explanation: EU MDR 2017/745 Chapter VII defines PMS and vigilance requirements enhancing lifecycle safety oversight. Option A mentions feedback but lacks full PMS detail, Option C covers design control, and D is non-device-specific. SubChapter: Regulatory Post-Market Surveillance
Q476. Answer: B
Explanation: SEM provides detailed surface imaging for fracture and microstructural analysis in failure investigations. FTIR and HPLC target chemical composition; XRF determines elemental content but lacks microfracture visualization. SubChapter: Failure Analysis
Q477. Answer: A
Explanation: TOC quantifies organic residue, verifying cleanliness prior to sterilization. Bioburden assesses microbial load post-cleaning, endotoxin tests detect pyrogens, and visual inspection lacks quantitative precision. SubChapter: Reprocessing Validation
Q478. Answer: A
Explanation: IEC 62304 Annex C aligns software risk management with ISO 14971 principles. Option B references general device risks, Option C covers planning, and D applies to cleanroom monitoring. SubChapter: Software Risk Management
Q479. Answer: A
Explanation: Half-cycle testing using biological indicators verifies sterilant penetration and lethality margin. Option B evaluates pyrogens, C gives process exposure only, and D misses microbial assurance. SubChapter: Sterilization Validation
Q480. Answer: C
Explanation: QFD translates user requirements into measurable design targets ensuring alignment during verification. DFMEA evaluates failure risks; Ishikawa and fishbone identify causes, not requirements translation. SubChapter: Design Verification
Q481. Answer: B
Explanation: The exceedance indicates environmental control failure requiring root-cause analysis and requalification per ISO 14644-2. Continuing or accepting deviations violates contamination-control principles; unverified filter replacement omits verification testing. SubChapter: Controlled Environments

Q482. Answer: A
Explanation: Labeling specifications reside in the DMR, which must be updated before production to maintain traceability. DHR records batch data, management reviews are strategic, and supplier files relate to procurement—not labeling control. SubChapter: Labeling and Documentation Control
Q483. Answer: A
Explanation: Thermometric mapping ensures consistent temperature and steam saturation throughout the load, verifying process uniformity. Biological and chemical indicators follow mapping; bioburden quantifies microbial load, not distribution uniformity. SubChapter: Sterilization Validation
Q484. Answer: B
Explanation: Strengthening insulation directly eliminates the hazard source per ISO 14971 risk-control hierarchy. Software lockouts and warnings are secondary barriers, and reduced inspection increases residual risk. SubChapter: Electrical Safety and Risk Management
Q485. Answer: A
Explanation: Section 820.30(f) mandates design-verification activities to confirm conformance with specified inputs. 820.70 addresses process control, 820.198 complaint handling, and 820.90 non-conforming product. SubChapter: Design Verification
Q486. Answer: C
Explanation: Class C denotes highest risk, where software failure may result in death or serious harm, requiring rigorous validation and documentation. Classes A and B correspond to negligible or non-serious outcomes; non-regulation is incorrect. SubChapter: Software Safety Classification
Q487. Answer: B
Explanation: Routine monitoring logs demonstrate maintained sterility assurance between revalidations. Protocols and IQs are one-time qualifications; supplier audits verify vendor compliance, not daily sterilization control. SubChapter: Sterilization Process Monitoring
Q488. Answer: B
Explanation: 21 CFR 801 governs device labeling accuracy and adequacy, including warnings and reuse instructions. ISO 13485 § 7.3.9 covers design transfer, 9001 is generic, and 820.184 addresses DHR content. SubChapter: Labeling Compliance
Q489. Answer: A
Explanation: Seal integrity defects require parameter optimization and full re-validation under ISO 11607 to ensure sterile barrier reliability. Continuing production or labeling changes ignores root cause; partial rejection lacks process control. SubChapter: Packaging Validation
Q490. Answer: B
Explanation: IEC 62366-1 integrates human-factors engineering with risk management to reduce use errors. ISO 14971 outlines general risk methodology, IEC 60601-1 covers electrical safety, and 9001 is non-device specific. SubChapter: Human Factors Engineering
Q491. Answer: C
Explanation: Missing sterilization records breach 21 CFR 820.180 record-retention and traceability obligations. DMR and validation documentation are upstream activities; design input is unrelated to lot-level traceability. SubChapter: Documentation and Traceability
Q492. Answer: A
Explanation: The Limulus Amebocyte Lysate (LAL) test detects bacterial endotoxins ensuring pyrogen-free status. TOC measures organic residue, bioburden counts microbes, and UV spectroscopy lacks specificity for endotoxins. SubChapter: Reprocessing Validation
Q493. Answer: A
Explanation: ISO 13485 acts as the harmonized foundation bridging QSR and MDR requirements globally. Dual or separate systems add redundancy; outsourcing does not ensure regulatory accountability. SubChapter: International Regulatory Integration

Q494. Answer: A
Explanation: IEC 62133 specifies safety requirements and tests for rechargeable batteries used in medical devices. ISO 14971 offers overall risk framework, 13485 defines QMS, 11135 covers EtO sterilization. SubChapter: Device Electrical Safety
Q495. Answer: B
Explanation: Performance Qualification (PQ) confirms process reproducibility under routine conditions, proving sterilization reliability. Installation verifies setup, design concerns equipment selection, and supplier qualification audits vendors. SubChapter: Sterilization Validation
Q496. Answer: C
Explanation: Cpk quantifies process capability relative to specification limits, crucial for verifying manufacturing consistency. Control charts monitor trends, regression predicts relationships, and Pareto prioritizes issues without quantifying capability. SubChapter: Process Capability Analysis
Q497. Answer: C
Explanation: ISO 14971 requires verifying control effectiveness and checking for unintended hazards after implementation. Analysis identifies hazards, evaluation compares acceptability, and design validation tests functional requirements. SubChapter: Risk Control Verification
Q498. Answer: B
Explanation: IEC 62366-1 emphasizes interface redesign to remove confusion rather than relying on labeling or training. Larger warnings and lockouts mitigate symptoms, not root cause. SubChapter: Human Factors Design
Q499. Answer: B
Explanation: Differential pressure mapping confirms directional air movement preventing contamination ingress. Airflow visualization illustrates flow patterns, particle counting measures contamination, and HEPA testing checks filter integrity. SubChapter: Controlled Environment Validation
Q500. Answer: A
Explanation: Setting alarms is a preventive control ensuring immediate detection of deviations before product impact. Corrective actions occur post-event; revalidation and supplier qualification address different lifecycle stages. SubChapter: Process Control and Monitoring

Questions (501-600)

Q501. A manufacturer must demonstrate reproducibility of sterilization results across three consecutive runs. Which validation stage applies?

A. Installation Qualification
B. Operational Qualification
C. Performance Qualification
D. Process Design Review

Q502. A risk assessment finds probability of patient harm = 1/10 000 and severity = serious. According to ISO 14971, this risk must be ___.

A. Automatically accepted
B. Evaluated for control or reduction
C. Ignored until complaints occur
D. Escalated only after market launch

Q503. Which test assesses particulate contamination from device packaging materials?

A. Bioburden test
B. Particulate shedding test
C. Endotoxin test
D. Burst strength test

Q504. A manufacturer develops an implant with a polymer coating. Which standard ensures evaluation of potential leachables?

A. ISO 10993-17
B. ISO 11137
C. ISO 14644
D. IEC 60601-1

Q505. A device's software controls dosage delivery. What is the most critical validation step?

A. User training documentation
B. Software hazard analysis and verification testing
C. Labeling review
D. Supplier audit of code repository

Q506. Which quality tool helps prioritize root causes when analyzing repeated device failures?

A. Pareto Chart
B. Scatter Diagram
C. Histogram
D. Run Chart

Q507. A cleanroom airflow visualization test shows turbulence near filling stations. What should the engineer implement first?

A. Stop production permanently
B. Identify and correct airflow imbalance
C. Increase gowning frequency
D. Replace sterilizer filters

Q508. Which document describes medical device QMS requirements for regulatory compliance?

A. ISO 9001
B. ISO 13485
C. ISO 14971
D. ISO 17025

Q509. A design control record lacks verification evidence for updated circuit boards. What risk does this create?

A. Loss of sterility
B. Non-conformance to design input requirements
C. Labeling misinterpretation
D. Process inefficiency
Q510. The engineer validates EtO residuals meet ISO 10993-7 limits. What is the primary purpose?
A. Confirm microbial lethality
B. Demonstrate biocompatibility of residual gases
C. Establish shelf life
D. Check labeling accuracy
Q511. What statistical tool identifies the most common defects in a manufacturing process?
A. Pareto Chart
B. Control Chart
C. Scatter Plot
D. Regression Analysis
Q512. A product uses sterile water in assembly. Which test verifies microbial control in utility systems?
A. Endotoxin testing
B. Total plate count
C. Conductivity test
D. Dissolved oxygen measurement
Q513. When a design team evaluates worst-case loading for sterilization, it is performing ___.
A. Installation Qualification
B. Operational Qualification
C. Performance Qualification
D. Design Validation
Q514. Which international standard defines requirements for medical electrical equipment safety?
A. IEC 60601-1
B. ISO 13485
C. ISO 11137
D. ISO 9001
Q515. A manufacturer introduces a new sterilization chamber. Which qualification step verifies correct installation before validation?
A. Installation Qualification
B. Operational Qualification
C. Performance Qualification
D. Process Validation
Q516. During risk management, new hazards are identified after design changes. What must be done per ISO 14971?
A. Close risk file and note changes
B. Re-evaluate risk analysis and controls
C. Ignore until next audit
D. Create separate file without review
Q517. Which test verifies HEPA filters maintain efficiency after installation?
A. Integrity (leak) test
B. Airflow velocity measurement
C. Particle count test
D. Air pressure balance test
Q518. For reusable devices, which validation proves the cleaning process removes protein residues to acceptable levels?

A. TOC and protein residue assays
B. Endotoxin testing only
C. Visual inspection
D. Microbial count only

Q519. A software anomaly occurs during device testing. What document must capture the issue per IEC 62304?

A. Risk management file
B. Software problem report
C. Design history file
D. Traceability matrix

Q520. Which sterilization method is most appropriate for heat-sensitive catheters?

A. Dry heat
B. Ethylene oxide (EtO) gas
C. Steam autoclaving
D. Gamma irradiation only

Q521. A design validation report for a surgical laser lacks temperature rise data on tissue. What requirement is violated?

A. Verification traceability
B. Validation under actual use conditions
C. Labeling accuracy
D. Supplier documentation control

Q522. Which document defines the regulatory basis for electronic records and signatures in medical device systems?

A. 21 CFR 820.70
B. 21 CFR 11
C. ISO 13485 § 4.2.4
D. ISO 9001 § 7.5

Q523. A packaging engineer evaluates tensile strength of sterile barrier seams. Which test standard applies?

A. ASTM F88
B. ISO 11135
C. ISO 10993
D. IEC 60601-1

Q524. After validation, a software update changes control logic. What must occur first per IEC 62304?

A. Continue using previous risk classification
B. Reassess and verify the change's impact
C. Document change after release only
D. Ignore minor updates

Q525. Which process ensures biological indicators achieve specified kill in radiation sterilization?

A. Dose audits
B. Half-cycle testing
C. Process challenge device placement
D. Endotoxin analysis

Q526. A design review reveals incomplete supplier qualification for a critical component. What must be done?

A. Issue deviation approval
B. Perform supplier audit and qualification
C. Proceed with production while monitoring

D. Ignore since component is non-sterile

Q527. Which ISO standard provides requirements for environmental control of cleanrooms?

A. ISO 11137-1

B. ISO 14644-1

C. ISO 13485 § 6.4

D. ISO 9001 § 8.2

Q528. During risk evaluation, the team cannot further reduce a hazard without impairing device function. ISO 14971 requires ___.

A. Eliminate the device design

B. Document risk-benefit analysis and justify acceptance

C. Transfer risk to user training

D. Cease production immediately

Q529. A reusable endoscope fails to achieve sterility after cleaning. What must be verified first?

A. Cleaning validation process parameters

B. User training records

C. Packaging integrity tests

D. Labeling instructions font size

Q530. Which standard defines requirements for risk management of electrical medical equipment?

A. ISO 14971

B. IEC 60601-1

C. ISO 13485

D. ISO 14644

Q531. A packaging process shows increasing seal defects. What is the most appropriate investigation tool?

A. Fishbone diagram

B. Scatter plot

C. Box-plot analysis

D. Histogram only

Q532. What is the primary purpose of using a "design traceability matrix"?

A. Track audit findings

B. Link design inputs to outputs and verification

C. Record training activities

D. Identify supplier performance

Q533. Which validation activity verifies process controls operate within established limits during qualification?

A. Operational Qualification (OQ)

B. Performance Qualification (PQ)

C. Installation Qualification (IQ)

D. Risk Evaluation

Q534. An audit finds a missing HEPA integrity test report. Which risk does this pose?

A. Increased sterilization temperature

B. Potential cleanroom contamination

C. Incorrect equipment labeling

D. Delayed shipment authorization

Q535. A design team uses Failure Mode and Effects Analysis (FMEA). The Risk Priority Number (RPN) is a product of ___.

A. Severity, Occurrence, Detection

B. Likelihood, Impact, Exposure

C. Frequency, Control, Verification
D. Hazard, Mitigation, Response

Q536. A validation engineer must confirm dose uniformity in gamma sterilization. Which tool is used?
A. Dosimeter mapping
B. Biological indicator placement
C. Endotoxin testing
D. Airflow visualization

Q537. Which standard covers risk management of in vitro diagnostic (IVD) medical devices?
A. ISO 14971
B. ISO 13485
C. ISO 20916
D. ISO 11135

Q538. In design transfer, what document ensures production uses approved specifications?
A. Device Master Record (DMR)
B. Device History Record (DHR)
C. Design History File (DHF)
D. Risk Management File (RMF)

Q539. A device uses radiation-sterilized components from a supplier. What evidence must the manufacturer obtain?
A. Supplier's dose validation report
B. Shipping temperature records
C. Calibration certificates only
D. Marketing approval letters

Q540. Which type of validation confirms device meets user needs under actual conditions of use?
A. Design Verification
B. Design Validation
C. Process Validation
D. Risk Evaluation

Q541. A post-market complaint revealed adhesive failure in a sterile package after shipment. What is the most appropriate corrective action?
A. Revise sterilization cycle
B. Conduct transportation simulation and seal strength re-validation
C. Update labeling only
D. Increase production quantity

Q542. During usability testing, users consistently press the wrong power button despite clear labels. What should the design team do?
A. Reinforce user training
B. Redesign interface layout per IEC 62366-1
C. Add warning decals
D. Reject user input data

Q543. A sterilization cycle produces over-lethal doses, degrading polymer components. What step ensures optimal cycle parameters?
A. Conduct process optimization study using half-cycle method
B. Reduce aeration time
C. Increase exposure pressure
D. Ignore degradation

Q544. A manufacturer integrates new firmware into an infusion pump. Which regulatory element must be updated?

A. Device Master Record
B. Software Problem Report
C. Design History File
D. Management Review Minutes

Q545. Which analytical tool quantifies relationship strength between sterilization temperature and microbial reduction?

A. Regression analysis
B. Pareto chart
C. Histogram
D. Box plot

Q546. A manufacturer adds new plasticizer to device housing. Which testing series ensures patient safety?

A. ISO 10993 biocompatibility evaluation
B. ISO 11137 dose mapping
C. ISO 14644 cleanroom classification
D. IEC 60601-1 performance test

Q547. Which metric demonstrates cleanroom recovery efficiency after disturbance?

A. Airflow velocity
B. Particle count recovery test
C. HEPA integrity test
D. Temperature mapping

Q548. A supplier provides pre-sterilized tubing. What must the manufacturer verify before use?

A. Supplier's sterilization validation report
B. Marketing authorization
C. Operator training record
D. Batch size agreement

Q549. What design-control document defines how verification activities will be performed?

A. Verification plan
B. Device History Record
C. Design Review Report
D. Management Review Summary

Q550. An autoclave validation reveals condensation on instruments. Which adjustment is most appropriate?

A. Extend drying phase and validate again
B. Increase load density
C. Skip equilibration time
D. Reduce vacuum cycles

Q551. Which requirement of ISO 13485 addresses environmental cleanliness and contamination control?

A. Clause 6.4
B. Clause 8.2.3
C. Clause 7.3.2
D. Clause 5.6.1

Q552. A failure analysis on an implant shows corrosion pits. Which method best determines elemental composition?

A. Infrared Spectroscopy (FTIR)
B. Differential Scanning Calorimetry (DSC)
C. High-Performance Liquid Chromatography (HPLC)

D. Energy-Dispersive X-ray Spectroscopy (EDS)

Q553. Which ISO document specifies requirements for radiation-sterilization dose establishment and validation?

A. ISO 11137-1
B. ISO 11135
C. ISO 13485
D. ISO 14644-1

Q554. A design change introduces new software module controlling temperature alarms. What must the team perform first?

A. Impact assessment and verification testing
B. Label revision
C. Complaint trend analysis
D. Production trial run

Q555. The risk-management file references outdated hazard data. What should the auditor require?

A. Risk file revision and current review
B. CAPA closure form
C. Updated marketing plan
D. Product recall notice

Q556. Which equipment qualification ensures utilities deliver required parameters before validation?

A. Installation Qualification
B. Operational Qualification
C. Performance Qualification
D. Design Qualification

Q557. A biocompatibility test reveals cytotoxicity. What is the most appropriate next step?

A. Update label precautions
B. Ignore since results are in vitro
C. Increase sterilization dose
D. Investigate materials and change composition

Q558. Which risk-analysis technique visually links hazards to their potential effects?

A. Fault Tree Analysis (FTA)
B. Control Chart
C. Scatter Diagram
D. Run Chart

Q559. Cleanroom certification found pressure differential below limits. What immediate action should be taken?

A. Investigate root cause and suspend production until restored
B. Continue production with documentation
C. Calibrate unrelated equipment
D. Increase personnel entry frequency

Q560. Which validation type confirms design specifications translate effectively into manufacturing processes?

A. Process Validation
B. Design Verification
C. Performance Qualification
D. Installation Qualification

Q561. During packaging validation, samples fail burst testing after humidity exposure. What corrective action is most appropriate?

A. Revise seal parameters and re-validate under worst conditions

B. Shorten sterilization exposure
C. Relabel humidity limits
D. Change box color

Q562. A software update introduces new alarm logic. What document must record verification results?

A. Supplier audit record
B. Design review minutes
C. Complaint log
D. Software verification report

Q563. A device shows recurring mechanical fractures. Which statistical tool best identifies the most frequent root cause?

A. Pareto chart
B. Scatter plot
C. Regression model
D. Run chart

Q564. Which ISO standard governs performance qualification for radiation sterilization?

A. ISO 11137-3
B. ISO 11135
C. ISO 14644-2
D. ISO 13485

Q565. An engineer confirms a cleanroom's airflow pattern with visible smoke. What is this test called?

A. Airflow visualization study
B. HEPA integrity test
C. Differential pressure mapping
D. Particle count verification

Q566. Risk analysis shows residual risk of electrical burn remains. What action aligns with ISO 14971?

A. Transfer risk to user training alone
B. Eliminate device entirely
C. Perform benefit–risk analysis and document acceptance
D. Ignore since probability is low

Q567. A new supplier provides sterilization services. Which initial activity is mandatory?

A. Supplier qualification audit
B. Final product sampling only
C. Process capability index review
D. Routine dose audit

Q568. Which design stage ensures manufacturing outputs are based on approved inputs and verifications?

A. Design transfer
B. Design planning
C. Design review
D. Risk evaluation

Q569. A manufacturer adds barcode UDI to labels. What benefit does this provide?

A. Traceability and post-market recall efficiency
B. Marketing appeal
C. Reduced manufacturing cost
D. Simpler sterilization cycle

Q570. What sterilization indicator verifies cycle parameters were met but not sterility assurance?

A. Bioburden test
B. Biological indicator

C. Endotoxin test
D. Chemical indicator

Q571. A device uses software to calculate dosage based on sensor input. Which validation step is most critical?

A. Software hazard analysis and verification testing
B. Label approval
C. Marketing evaluation
D. Operator training plan

Q572. Which test verifies the effectiveness of equipment cleaning before sterilization?

A. TOC and protein residue assay
B. Endotoxin test only
C. Color indicator label
D. Visual inspection alone

Q573. Which statistical index evaluates if a process can meet specifications consistently?

A. Cpk
B. RPN
C. p-value
D. t-score

Q574. During gamma sterilization validation, the lowest dose still achieving sterility is determined. What term describes this?

A. Sub-lethal dose
B. Challenge dose
C. Verification dose
D. Screening dose

Q575. Which standard provides guidance for human-factors validation testing?

A. IEC 62366-1
B. ISO 14971
C. ISO 9001
D. ISO 13485

Q576. Which method detects surface residues on sterilized equipment after EtO cycles?

A. Gas chromatography analysis
B. UV-Vis spectrophotometry
C. Endotoxin test
D. Microbial swab test

Q577. A design review finds risk controls not verified as effective. What must occur next?

A. Perform risk-control verification testing
B. Close risk file as is
C. Update marketing brochure
D. Initiate post-market reporting

Q578. Which cleanroom parameter directly controls particulate infiltration between zones?

A. Lighting intensity
B. Relative humidity
C. Pressure differential
D. Noise level

Q579. Which validation phase verifies a process operates effectively under routine production conditions?

A. Performance Qualification (PQ)
B. Operational Qualification (OQ)

C. Installation Qualification (IQ)
D. Design Qualification (DQ)

Q580. A company introduces new ethylene oxide sterilizer software. What combined validation is required?
A. Software and process validation
B. Labeling and design verification
C. Risk evaluation only
D. Supplier qualification

Q581. A manufacturer introduces a 3-D-printed orthopedic implant. Before commercial release, which validation step ensures reproducibility across different printers?
A. Process validation using representative machines
B. Prototype verification only
C. Supplier declaration review
D. Visual inspection of samples

Q582. An AI-driven diagnostic device adapts algorithms using real-world data. Which regulatory principle ensures ongoing software safety?
A. Labeling warning expansion
B. Fixed algorithm lock post-approval
C. Manual operator overrides only
D. Continuous learning change-control and re-validation plan

Q583. Which test demonstrates that a sterilized implant maintains mechanical strength after five-year accelerated aging?
A. Post-aging tensile and fatigue testing
B. Visual inspection only
C. Bioburden enumeration
D. Software verification

Q584. A cybersecurity review of a wireless insulin pump identifies unencrypted data transfer. What corrective measure best mitigates the risk?
A. Implement end-to-end encryption and penetration testing
B. Add a new label cautioning network risk
C. Restrict sales temporarily
D. Increase sampling frequency

Q585. During design transfer of a catheter line, which documentation ensures correct process parameters are used in production?
A. Device Master Record
B. Design History File
C. Audit plan
D. Risk management report

Q586. A biologics-device combination product uses polymer coating to control drug release. Which validation confirms uniform coating thickness?
A. Supplier certificate reliance
B. Visual comparison of color
C. Batch record review only
D. Process validation using statistical sampling and coating-weight analysis

Q587. An engineer must demonstrate that reprocessed single-use instruments are equivalent to new ones. Which study supports this claim?
A. Comparative performance and material integrity testing after multiple cycles
B. Supplier qualification audit

C. Label readability test
D. Operator training evaluation

Q588. A robotic surgical system relies on motion-control sensors. What verification ensures patient-safety tolerance limits are met?
A. Sensor calibration and accuracy verification under load
B. User interface simulation
C. Cleaning validation
D. Post-market surveillance only

Q589. When auditing sterilization of single-use syringes, which document defines microbial load-reduction acceptance criteria?
A. ISO 11737-1 bioburden standard
B. ISO 11135 sterilization standard
C. ISO 13485 clause 8.2
D. ISO 14644-3 test method

Q590. A design engineer evaluates additive-manufactured implants for internal voids. Which technology is most appropriate?
A. V
B. Optical microscopy only
C. Density weighing
D. Computed tomography (CT) nondestructive inspection

Q591. A developer integrates a cloud-based mobile app to display diagnostic data. Which control ensures data integrity and privacy?
A. Implementation of validated encryption and access control per HIPAA
B. Adding extra color indicators
C. Disabling all cloud functions
D. Increasing app download limits

Q592. A validation engineer must verify that UV sterilization effectively inactivates bacteria on flexible endoscopes. Which evidence is required?
A. Microbial log-reduction data under worst-case conditions
B. Visual inspection for cleanliness
C. Lamp output calibration alone
D. Documentation of operator training

Q593. A nanomaterial-coated stent raises concerns about particulate release. Which test should be performed?
A. Particle-shedding and leachables testing in simulated-use conditions
B. Tensile strength testing only
C. Accelerated aging test
D. Label legibility inspection

Q594. Which approach demonstrates that an AI image-analysis tool maintains accuracy across patient populations?
A. Algorithm code review
B. Single-site retrospective testing
C. Developer internal verification only
D. Validation using diverse, representative datasets and performance metrics

Q595. A company adopts single-use bioprocess bags for sterile filtration. Which qualification verifies compatibility with product contact fluids?
A. Extractables and leachables study under simulated use
B. Container-closure integrity test only

C. Label aging test
D. Visual inspection after use
Q596. Which standard provides guidance for integration of usability engineering into medical-device design?
A. IEC 62366-1
B. ISO 13485
C. ISO 9001
D. ISO 11137-2
Q597. A connected home-use glucose monitor communicates via Bluetooth. Which validation is critical before release?
A. Wireless coexistence and cybersecurity testing per FDA guidance
B. End-user labeling review
C. Temperature conditioning
D. Production line sampling
Q598. What verification demonstrates that manufacturing equipment produces consistent dimensional tolerances for orthopedic screws?
A. Training records review
B. Supplier audit
C. Packaging validation
D. Gauge repeatability and reproducibility (GR&R) study
Q599. A manufacturer deploys blockchain for device-traceability. What validation element ensures compliance with QMS requirements?
A. Verification of data immutability, audit trails, and access control
B. Proof-of-stake algorithm documentation only
C. Employee blockchain training records
D. Marketing approval certificate
Q600. A post-market field failure shows sensor drift in AI-based patient monitors. Which follow-up is required?
A. Root-cause investigation and model re-training validation
B. User training reissue
C. Cosmetic design update
D. Production rate increase

Answer key and Explanation (501-600)

Q501. Answer: C
Explanation: Performance Qualification verifies that a validated process consistently produces sterile output under routine conditions across multiple cycles. Installation checks setup; Operational tests parameters; Design Review concerns planning, not production consistency. SubChapter: Sterilization Validation
Q502. Answer: B
Explanation: ISO 14971 requires assessing even low-probability serious harms for additional control or reduction to ensure acceptability. Automatic acceptance or deferral violates proactive risk management principles. SubChapter: Risk Evaluation
Q503. Answer: B
Explanation: Particulate shedding tests measure particles released from packaging to ensure compliance with cleanliness standards. Bioburden quantifies microbes, endotoxin detects pyrogens, and burst testing measures seal integrity. SubChapter: Packaging Cleanliness Validation
Q504. Answer: A
Explanation: ISO 10993-17 provides toxicological risk assessment for leachables and extractables from device materials. ISO 11137 covers sterilization, 14644 cleanrooms, and 60601-1 electrical safety. SubChapter: Biocompatibility and Toxicology
Q505. Answer: B
Explanation: For safety-critical software, hazard analysis and verification testing confirm functional accuracy and fail-safe performance per IEC 62304 Class C. Training, labeling, or supplier audits cannot replace direct validation. SubChapter: Software Validation
Q506. Answer: A
Explanation: Pareto Charts rank failure causes by frequency, focusing corrective actions on the vital few contributors. Scatter, histogram, and run charts describe relationships or distributions without prioritization. SubChapter: Failure Analysis Tools
Q507. Answer: B
Explanation: Correcting airflow imbalance restores laminar flow protecting sterile zones, as required by ISO 14644-3. Stopping production may be excessive, and other options address unrelated contamination sources. SubChapter: Controlled Environment Qualification
Q508. Answer: B
Explanation: ISO 13485 specifies comprehensive QMS requirements tailored to medical devices and regulatory alignment. ISO 9001 is generic, 14971 covers risk management, and 17025 applies to test laboratories. SubChapter: Quality Management System Framework
Q509. Answer: B
Explanation: Missing verification evidence breaks the traceability chain proving design outputs meet inputs, violating 21 CFR 820.30(f). The other risks are secondary or unrelated. SubChapter: Design Verification
Q510. Answer: B
Explanation: ISO 10993-7 sets acceptable EtO residual levels to protect patients from toxic exposure, confirming biocompatibility. Microbial lethality and shelf life are separate validations; labeling is unrelated. SubChapter: Sterilization Residue Safety
Q511. Answer: A
Explanation: The Pareto Chart quickly highlights the few defects responsible for most problems, supporting focused corrective action. Control and scatter charts analyze variation trends; regression predicts relationships. SubChapter: Quality Improvement Tools
Q512. Answer: B

Explanation: Total plate count confirms microbial control within purified water systems as required by ISO and FDA guidelines. Endotoxin, conductivity, and oxygen tests measure other parameters not overall bioburden. SubChapter: Utilities and Environmental Monitoring

Q513. Answer: B

Explanation: Operational Qualification verifies process control under defined extremes, including worst-case loads, to ensure parameters meet acceptance criteria. Installation verifies equipment setup; Performance ensures routine reproducibility; Design Validation tests final product. SubChapter: Sterilization Validation

Q514. Answer: A

Explanation: IEC 60601-1 sets fundamental safety and essential performance requirements for medical electrical devices. ISO 13485 covers QMS, 11137 sterilization, and 9001 generic quality systems. SubChapter: Electrical Safety

Q515. Answer: A

Explanation: Installation Qualification confirms equipment is installed per specifications and operates within defined parameters before process validation. Operational and Performance follow sequentially; process validation finalizes control. SubChapter: Equipment Qualification

Q516. Answer: B

Explanation: ISO 14971 requires updating risk analysis to reflect design changes and assessing new hazards for adequate control. Closing or ignoring files violates the continuous risk management cycle. SubChapter: Risk Management Maintenance

Q517. Answer: A

Explanation: HEPA integrity tests detect leaks and confirm filter performance meets ISO 14644-3 requirements. Velocity and pressure tests support flow balance; particle counts monitor environment but not filter integrity. SubChapter: Cleanroom Qualification

Q518. Answer: A

Explanation: TOC and protein assays quantify organic residues, demonstrating cleaning effectiveness for reusable devices per FDA and ISO guidelines. Endotoxin or microbial tests alone lack completeness; visual inspection is insufficient. SubChapter: Reprocessing Validation

Q519. Answer: B

Explanation: IEC 62304 requires documenting anomalies in software problem reports to ensure tracking and resolution. Risk files record hazards; history files cover entire design; traceability links requirements to tests. SubChapter: Software Maintenance

Q520. Answer: B

Explanation: EtO sterilization effectively processes heat- and moisture-sensitive materials without damaging catheters. Dry heat and steam exceed temperature tolerance; gamma can degrade polymers. SubChapter: Sterilization Method Selection

Q521. Answer: B

Explanation: Design validation must confirm device performance under simulated or actual conditions, including heat impact on tissue. Missing such data means incomplete validation. Verification traceability and labeling are separate controls, while supplier documentation is unrelated. SubChapter: Design Validation

Q522. Answer: B

Explanation: 21 CFR 11 governs FDA requirements for electronic records and signatures to ensure authenticity, integrity, and confidentiality. 820.70 concerns process control, ISO 13485 § 4.2.4 covers records retention, and 9001 § 7.5 relates to documentation but not regulatory e-signatures. SubChapter: Regulatory Compliance

Q523. Answer: A

Explanation: ASTM F88 measures seal tensile strength ensuring sterile barrier reliability. ISO 11135 covers EtO sterilization, ISO 10993 addresses biocompatibility, and IEC 60601-1 applies to electrical safety. SubChapter: Packaging Validation

Q524. Answer: B

Explanation: IEC 62304 mandates impact assessment and re-verification of any software change before release. Ignoring or post-documenting violates lifecycle integrity; risk class may also change depending on update scope. SubChapter: Software Maintenance and Change Control

Q525. Answer: C

Explanation: Process challenge devices verify dose penetration and BI exposure during sterilization, ensuring lethality validation. Dose audits occur post-validation; half-cycles apply mainly to EtO; endotoxin analysis checks pyrogens, not sterility. SubChapter: Sterilization Validation

Q526. Answer: B

Explanation: Critical suppliers must be audited and qualified to ensure component reliability and regulatory compliance. Deviations or monitoring without qualification risk nonconformance; non-sterile status does not negate criticality. SubChapter: Supplier Quality Management

Q527. Answer: B

Explanation: ISO 14644-1 classifies cleanrooms by airborne particulate concentrations, guiding design and monitoring. ISO 11137 covers sterilization, 13485 § 6.4 mentions infrastructure broadly, and 9001 is non-specific. SubChapter: Controlled Environment Standards

Q528. Answer: B

Explanation: When further reduction is impossible, ISO 14971 permits risk acceptance if benefit outweighs residual risk and is documented. Eliminating design or shifting risk without justification breaches compliance. SubChapter: Residual Risk Assessment

Q529. Answer: A

Explanation: Ineffective sterility often results from poor cleaning; verifying validated parameters ensures biofilm removal before sterilization. Training and labels are secondary; packaging integrity is post-sterilization. SubChapter: Reprocessing Validation

Q530. Answer: B

Explanation: IEC 60601-1 integrates risk management from ISO 14971 specifically for medical electrical equipment safety and performance. ISO 14971 is general; 13485 covers QMS; 14644 applies to cleanrooms. SubChapter: Electrical Safety

Q531. Answer: A

Explanation: Fishbone (Ishikawa) diagrams help identify potential root causes across categories like materials, methods, machines, and environment. Other charts show data distributions but lack causal analysis. SubChapter: Failure Investigation

Q532. Answer: B

Explanation: A traceability matrix ensures each design input has corresponding output and verification evidence, maintaining compliance with 21 CFR 820.30. Audit, training, and supplier records are managed elsewhere. SubChapter: Design Control Documentation

Q533. Answer: A

Explanation: OQ tests process control parameters to ensure they consistently achieve expected outcomes before PQ. IQ verifies setup; PQ evaluates routine performance; risk evaluation is analytical. SubChapter: Process Qualification

Q534. Answer: B

Explanation: Without HEPA integrity records, airborne contamination risk rises, compromising product sterility. Other options do not directly stem from missing test documentation. SubChapter: Controlled Environment Monitoring

Q535. Answer: A

Explanation: RPN = Severity × Occurrence × Detection quantifies risk for prioritizing mitigation actions. Other sets describe risk generically but don't match FMEA structure. SubChapter: Risk Analysis Techniques

Q536. Answer: A

Explanation: Dosimeter mapping quantifies radiation distribution to ensure uniform dose delivery throughout the load. BI placement verifies lethality but not dose spread; other tests address unrelated parameters. SubChapter: Sterilization Validation

Q537. Answer: C

Explanation: ISO 20916 applies risk and performance requirements to in vitro diagnostic medical devices. ISO 14971 is general; 13485 defines QMS; 11135 relates to EtO sterilization. SubChapter: IVD Regulatory Standards

Q538. Answer: A

Explanation: DMR contains approved specifications, procedures, and drawings for manufacture, ensuring design-to-production consistency. DHR records batch data; DHF shows design evidence; RMF documents risks. SubChapter: Design Transfer

Q539. Answer: A

Explanation: Manufacturers must verify supplier sterilization validation data for compliance with ISO 11137 requirements. Shipping and calibration data support other controls; marketing letters are non-technical. SubChapter: Supplier Process Validation

Q540. Answer: B

Explanation: Design validation tests finished devices in real or simulated use to ensure user needs are met per 21 CFR 820.30(g). Verification checks inputs; process validation ensures manufacturing consistency; risk evaluation assesses hazards. SubChapter: Design Validation

Q541. Answer: B

Explanation: Transit stress can weaken seals; therefore, ISTA transportation simulation and seal-strength re-validation under ISO 11607 confirm packaging robustness. Adjusting sterilization or labeling ignores the true cause, while higher output risks further failures. SubChapter: Packaging Validation

Q542. Answer: B

Explanation: IEC 62366-1 requires eliminating design-induced errors by modifying interface layout, shape, or feedback mechanisms. Training and warnings treat symptoms, not root cause; discarding feedback violates human-factors practice. SubChapter: Human Factors Engineering

Q543. Answer: A

Explanation: Half-cycle studies determine minimal effective dose, balancing sterility assurance with material compatibility. Reducing aeration or raising pressure can worsen degradation; ignoring issues violates validation integrity. SubChapter: Sterilization Process Optimization

Q544. Answer: C

Explanation: The Design History File documents all design changes, including firmware updates, per 21 CFR 820.30(j). Master Records control production specs, while problem reports handle anomalies only. SubChapter: Design Documentation Control

Q545. Answer: A

Explanation: Regression analysis determines correlation and predictive relationship between temperature and microbial log-reduction, supporting validation modeling. Pareto prioritizes causes, histograms and box plots display distributions without correlation quantification. SubChapter: Statistical Analysis in Validation

Q546. Answer: A

Explanation: ISO 10993 testing confirms material cytotoxicity, sensitization, and systemic safety after formulation change. Dose mapping, cleanroom, or electrical standards address unrelated parameters. SubChapter: Biocompatibility

Q547. Answer: B
Explanation: Recovery testing measures time to restore particulate levels post-disturbance, reflecting ventilation performance. Velocity shows speed but not recovery; integrity and temperature tests serve different purposes. SubChapter: Controlled Environment Monitoring
Q548. Answer: A
Explanation: Verification of supplier's validated sterilization process ensures sterility assurance compliance with ISO 11137. Marketing or training documents do not confirm process adequacy; batch size is contractual. SubChapter: Supplier Process Validation
Q549. Answer: A
Explanation: A verification plan details methods, acceptance criteria, and responsibilities for confirming design outputs meet inputs per 21 CFR 820.30(f). Other documents record outcomes or management oversight, not execution planning. SubChapter: Design Verification
Q550. Answer: A
Explanation: Extending drying phase eliminates residual moisture ensuring sterile barrier maintenance. Increasing density or skipping equilibration worsens results; fewer vacuum cycles impair steam penetration. SubChapter: Steam Sterilization Validation
Q551. Answer: A
Explanation: Clause 6.4 mandates controlling work environment conditions to prevent contamination of product. Clause 8.2.3 covers monitoring, 7.3.2 design inputs, and 5.6.1 management reviews. SubChapter: Environmental Control Requirements
Q552. Answer: D
Explanation: EDS identifies elemental makeup at corrosion sites, revealing contamination or alloy defects. DSC measures thermal transitions, HPLC and FTIR analyze organics, unsuitable for metal analysis. SubChapter: Failure Analysis
Q553. Answer: A
Explanation: ISO 11137-1 defines validation, routine control, and dose-establishment for radiation sterilization. ISO 11135 governs EtO, 13485 QMS, and 14644 cleanrooms. SubChapter: Radiation Sterilization Validation
Q554. Answer: A
Explanation: Any software modification requires documented impact assessment and verification before release per IEC 62304. Label or complaint updates occur later; production trials risk unvalidated operation. SubChapter: Software Change Control
Q555. Answer: A
Explanation: ISO 14971 mandates maintaining current risk documentation reflecting latest post-market information; outdated files compromise safety evidence. CAPA and recall are separate responses, marketing plans unrelated. SubChapter: Risk File Maintenance
Q556. Answer: A
Explanation: Installation Qualification confirms utilities and instruments are installed, calibrated, and functioning within design specifications before OQ and PQ. Later stages test performance, not installation. SubChapter: Equipment Qualification
Q557. Answer: D
Explanation: Cytotoxicity indicates material incompatibility; composition review and reformulation ensure patient safety. Ignoring, over-sterilizing, or labeling cannot mitigate intrinsic material toxicity. SubChapter: Biocompatibility Evaluation
Q558. Answer: A
Explanation: FTA maps logical relationships between root causes and adverse events, supporting proactive risk mitigation. Control, scatter, and run charts analyze data trends but not causal logic. SubChapter: Risk Analysis Tools

Q559. Answer: A
Explanation: Loss of pressure differential risks contamination; production must pause until cause is corrected and qualification restored per ISO 14644-2. Continuing operation violates contamination-control standards. SubChapter: Controlled Environment Response
Q560. Answer: A
Explanation: Process Validation demonstrates that manufacturing consistently produces product meeting design specifications under routine conditions. Verification checks inputs; PQ tests specific runs; IQ verifies setup. SubChapter: Process Validation
Q561. Answer: A
Explanation: Moisture weakens seals; revising sealing temperature, pressure, or dwell time and re-validating ensures barrier strength per ISO 11607. Relabeling or cosmetic changes don't solve failure; sterilization time rarely affects humidity-driven seal weakness. SubChapter: Packaging Validation
Q562. Answer: D
Explanation: Verification reports document objective evidence that revised code performs as intended under IEC 62304. Design reviews summarize discussion, complaint logs capture post-market issues, and supplier audits verify vendor compliance. SubChapter: Software Verification
Q563. Answer: A
Explanation: The Pareto chart ranks failure modes by frequency, revealing dominant contributors for prioritized action. Scatter, regression, and run charts describe relationships or time trends without highlighting major categories. SubChapter: Failure Analysis Tools
Q564. Answer: A
Explanation: ISO 11137-3 provides detailed guidance for performance qualification and ongoing dose monitoring of radiation sterilization. ISO 11135 covers EtO, 14644 environmental cleanrooms, and 13485 general QMS requirements. SubChapter: Radiation Sterilization
Q565. Answer: A
Explanation: Airflow visualization uses smoke to observe laminar flow and identify turbulence around critical zones as required by ISO 14644-3. Integrity, pressure, and particle tests measure different environmental parameters. SubChapter: Controlled Environment Qualification
Q566. Answer: C
Explanation: ISO 14971 requires documented benefit–risk justification when residual risk cannot be further reduced. Elimination may not be feasible; training alone is insufficient, and ignoring risk violates policy. SubChapter: Residual Risk Evaluation
Q567. Answer: A
Explanation: Before use, a qualification audit verifies supplier compliance with ISO 11137 or 11135 and QMS requirements. Sampling or dose audits occur after approval; capability indices alone don't prove compliance. SubChapter: Supplier Quality Management
Q568. Answer: A
Explanation: Design transfer converts approved design data into production specifications, ensuring manufacturing accuracy per 21 CFR 820.30. Planning organizes tasks, reviews evaluate progress, and risk analysis addresses safety aspects. SubChapter: Design Transfer
Q569. Answer: A
Explanation: UDI system enhances traceability through supply chain and supports effective recalls and post-market surveillance. Marketing and cost benefits are secondary; sterilization is unrelated. SubChapter: Labeling and UDI
Q570. Answer: D
Explanation: Chemical indicators react to temperature, time, or gas exposure, confirming cycle achievement without proving microbial kill. Biological indicators verify lethality; endotoxin and bioburden tests serve different purposes. SubChapter: Sterilization Monitoring

Q571. Answer: A
Explanation: Software controlling dosage must undergo hazard analysis and verification to ensure accuracy per IEC 62304 and ISO 14971. Labeling and training are secondary risk controls. SubChapter: Software Validation
Q572. Answer: A
Explanation: TOC and protein assays quantify organic residues to confirm cleaning efficacy for reusable devices. Endotoxin testing and visual inspection are partial methods and insufficient alone. SubChapter: Reprocessing Validation
Q573. Answer: A
Explanation: Cpk (capability index) quantifies how well process output fits within spec limits, guiding validation decisions. RPN applies to risk priority, p-value and t-score relate to hypothesis tests. SubChapter: Process Capability Analysis
Q574. Answer: C
Explanation: Verification dose is the minimum validated radiation dose that achieves required Sterility Assurance Level per ISO 11137. Other terms describe experimental or non-standard conditions. SubChapter: Radiation Sterilization
Q575. Answer: A
Explanation: IEC 62366-1 specifies methods to evaluate user interaction and reduce use errors through usability validation. ISO 14971 covers risk framework, 13485 QMS, and 9001 generic quality management. SubChapter: Human Factors Engineering
Q576. Answer: A
Explanation: Gas chromatography quantifies EtO residuals on materials, verifying compliance with ISO 10993-7 limits. UV-Vis and microbial tests address other properties; endotoxin testing targets biological contaminants. SubChapter: Residual Gas Testing
Q577. Answer: A
Explanation: ISO 14971 requires verifying risk-control effectiveness through testing or analysis before closure. Skipping verification or marketing updates fails compliance; post-market steps occur after release. SubChapter: Risk Control Verification
Q578. Answer: C
Explanation: Maintaining positive pressure differentials prevents contaminant migration between zones per ISO 14644-2. Humidity and lighting affect comfort, not containment; noise is irrelevant to particulate control. SubChapter: Environmental Control
Q579. Answer: A
Explanation: PQ confirms process consistency and output quality during normal production after IQ and OQ are complete. OQ tests control ranges; IQ verifies setup; DQ defines requirements. SubChapter: Process Validation
Q580. Answer: A
Explanation: Software controlling sterilization must be validated with the process to demonstrate accuracy and safety per IEC 62304 and ISO 11135. Labeling, risk review, or supplier qualification alone are insufficient. SubChapter: Software-Integrated Process Validation
Q581. Answer: A
Explanation: Process validation across representative printers confirms consistent mechanical properties and biocompatibility regardless of equipment variation. Prototype checks or declarations don't prove reproducibility, and visual inspection can't assess internal defects. This aligns with ISO/ASTM 52920 additive-manufacturing process qualification. SubChapter: Additive Manufacturing Validation
Q582. Answer: D
Explanation: FDA's Good Machine Learning Practice (GMLP) and IEC 62304 require lifecycle controls for adaptive algorithms, including documented re-validation after model updates. Locking algorithms limits

improvement, and labeling or overrides cannot maintain performance assurance. SubChapter: Artificial Intelligence in Medical Devices

Q583. Answer: A

Explanation: Accelerated-aging studies followed by mechanical testing confirm that long-term packaging and sterilization do not degrade device integrity. Visual or microbial tests miss structural changes, and software verification is irrelevant. SubChapter: Shelf-Life and Packaging Stability

Q584. Answer: A

Explanation: FDA pre- and post-market cybersecurity guidance and IEC 81001-5-1 emphasize encryption, authentication, and security validation to prevent exploitation. Label warnings or temporary sales holds don't remediate systemic vulnerability; sampling doesn't address software threats. SubChapter: Cybersecurity Risk Management

Q585. Answer: A

Explanation: The Device Master Record details approved drawings, materials, and validated process parameters controlling production. The Design History File contains development evidence; audits and risk reports serve different purposes. SubChapter: Design Transfer Documentation

Q586. Answer: D

Explanation: Quantitative coating-weight and thickness validation demonstrates uniform drug distribution, meeting FDA combination-product requirements. Visual or documentation checks alone cannot assure consistency or performance. SubChapter: Combination Product Validation

Q587. Answer: A

Explanation: Comparative validation under FDA 21 CFR 820 and ISO 17664 shows that cleaning, sterilization, and reuse don't compromise function or materials. Other options fail to prove equivalence or durability. SubChapter: Reprocessing Validation

Q588. Answer: A

Explanation: Calibration and accuracy verification confirm sensor output within specified tolerances, preventing hazardous motion. Interface simulation or surveillance detect issues later; cleaning validation is unrelated. IEC 60601-1 and IEC 80601-2-77 provide performance guidance. SubChapter: Robotics and Mechatronic Validation

Q589. Answer: A

Explanation: ISO 11737-1 specifies methods for bioburden determination and acceptance criteria prior to sterilization validation. ISO 11135 defines process parameters, 13485 concerns QMS, and 14644 covers environment testing. SubChapter: Bioburden Determination

Q590. Answer: D

Explanation: CT scanning provides 3-D nondestructive analysis of internal geometry and porosity, ensuring structural integrity in 3-D-printed devices. Microscopy, weighing, and thermal scans cannot detect deep voids effectively. SubChapter: Additive Manufacturing Quality Control

Q591. Answer: A

Explanation: Encryption, authentication, and HIPAA-compliant access validation maintain data confidentiality and integrity for medical apps, per FDA cybersecurity and IEC 81001-5-1 guidance. Cosmetic or operational adjustments provide no security assurance. SubChapter: Digital Health Data Security

Q592. Answer: A

Explanation: Demonstrating ≥6-log microbial reduction under worst-case load and geometry confirms process effectiveness per ISO 15858 and FDA guidance. Visual checks or calibration alone cannot assure sterility. SubChapter: Alternative Sterilization Technologies

Q593. Answer: A

Explanation: Simulated-use particle-shedding and extractables studies determine nanoparticle stability and potential patient exposure, complying with ISO 10993-18 and FDA nanomaterial guidance. Mechanical or labeling tests miss this hazard. SubChapter: Nanomaterials Safety Evaluation

Q594. Answer: D

Explanation: Broad, representative validation datasets prevent algorithmic bias and confirm consistent diagnostic accuracy per FDA GMLP principles. Limited or internal tests lack generalizability; code reviews don't measure output accuracy. SubChapter: AI/ML Validation

Q595. Answer: A

Explanation: Extractables and leachables studies identify potential chemical migration into fluids, ensuring material compatibility. Integrity or visual tests confirm sealing but not chemical safety; labeling checks are unrelated. SubChapter: Material Compatibility Validation

Q596. Answer: A

Explanation: IEC 62366-1 details usability engineering processes ensuring safe and effective device interaction, including user testing and risk mitigation. ISO 13485 covers QMS, 9001 generic quality, and 11137 sterilization. SubChapter: Human Factors Engineering

Q597. Answer: A

Explanation: Wireless coexistence testing verifies reliable data transmission amidst interference, while cybersecurity validation ensures data protection, satisfying FDA and ANSI C63.27 recommendations. Label or environmental tests don't ensure connectivity integrity. SubChapter: Connected Device Validation

Q598. Answer: D

Explanation: GR&R analysis quantifies measurement system variation, confirming process control precision for dimensional attributes. Audits, packaging, or training do not provide quantitative measurement capability data. SubChapter: Metrology and Process Control

Q599. Answer: A

Explanation: Validating immutability, traceability, and secure access demonstrates that blockchain maintains record integrity per ISO 13485 and 21 CFR 820.180. Other elements lack direct compliance assurance. SubChapter: Emerging Digital Technologies

Q600. Answer: A

Explanation: Investigating sensor drift and validating re-trained AI model ensures maintained diagnostic accuracy, fulfilling ISO 14971 and GMLP expectations. Training or cosmetic changes don't correct algorithmic deviation; increasing production worsens risk exposure. SubChapter: Post-Market Algorithm Maintenance

Questions (601-700)

Q601. A new sterilizer software automatically adjusts pressure levels. What validation ensures reliable automation?

A. Functional test runs
B. Simulated cycle test
C. Performance validation
D. Software verification

Q602. An additive manufacturing engineer changes build orientation for implants. What study confirms product consistency?

A. Mechanical testing study
B. Thermal stress test
C. Porosity scan test
D. Powder flow test

Q603. A cybersecurity audit finds open network ports on a pacemaker programmer. What must the manufacturer do?

A. Patch and verify
B. Report and wait
C. Reboot device
D. Disable Wi-Fi

Q604. Which standard governs risk management integration in design processes?

A. ISO 14971
B. ISO 11137
C. ISO 14644
D. ISO 10993

Q605. A manufacturer introduces cloud connectivity for patient devices. What is a required validation?

A. Product color check
B. User comfort survey
C. Data transfer security
D. Training attendance

Q606. Which test determines sterilization load placement efficiency?

A. Heat penetration test
B. Pressure leak test
C. Humidity test
D. Label adhesion test

Q607. During usability evaluation, users confuse power and reset buttons. What correction ensures safety?

A. Redesign layout
B. Add text note
C. Increase brightness
D. Extend training

Q608. What tool confirms measuring device precision across operators?

A. GR&R study
B. FMEA table
C. Pareto chart
D. Control chart

Q609. A robot-assisted surgical arm fails accuracy testing. What must be validated again?

A. Cable routing

B. Software interface
C. Power supply
D. Position calibration

Q610. Which document outlines approved design changes for production?
A. Change request log
B. Management review note
C. Supplier invoice copy
D. Maintenance checklist

Q611. A cleaning process validation shows protein residues. What is the next best action?
A. Adjust cleaning time
B. Discard equipment
C. Change packaging
D. Ignore deviation

Q612. A 3D-printed dental tool exhibits unexpected porosity. What corrective validation should follow?
A. Density mapping
B. Fatigue testing
C. Electrical test
D. Leak test

Q613. Which ISO standard defines medical electrical safety?
A. ISO 9001
B. ISO 13485
C. ISO 11137
D. IEC 60601

Q614. What activity ensures sterilization dose remains valid over time?
A. Dose audit
B. Visual check
C. Label update
D. Weight test

Q615. Which process monitors airborne particles in cleanrooms?
A. Particle counting
B. Light scanning
C. Noise sampling
D. Color coding

Q616. A risk analysis identifies residual data-security hazards. What is required?
A. Justify acceptance
B. Ignore finding
C. Stop all work
D. Extend training

Q617. A lab upgrades sensors for temperature mapping. What must be verified?
A. Audit readiness
B. Operator skill
C. Data label design
D. Calibration accuracy

Q618. What evidence supports equivalence of a reprocessed catheter to new product?
A. Performance test data
B. Label design check
C. Operator certificate

D. Batch count sheet

Q619. A developer integrates an AI triage system in diagnostic software. What must be confirmed?

A. Algorithm accuracy
B. Device label font
C. Battery connector
D. Packaging layout

Q620. Which qualification step verifies utilities meet installation design criteria?

A. IQ stage
B. PQ stage
C. OQ stage
D. DQ stage

Q621. A sterilization audit finds no record of chamber temperature calibration. What action restores compliance?

A. Replace label
B. Add note only
C. Delay shipment
D. Calibrate sensor

Q622. A new coating process changes implant friction properties. What study verifies performance?

A. Wear testing
B. Visual check
C. Supplier form
D. Label audit

Q623. Engineers introduce a robotic inspection system for assembly lines. What must be proven first?

A. Detection accuracy
B. Speed rating
C. Power draw
D. Paint finish

Q624. A supplier modifies polymer resin composition. What qualification step is needed?

A. Biocompatibility retest
B. Label update
C. Invoice review
D. Audit waiver

Q625. A smart inhaler transmits dose data to an app. What verification ensures proper transfer?

A. Shelf labeling
B. Color consistency
C. Shipping check
D. Connectivity test

Q626. A packaging engineer evaluates sterile barrier peel force. Which test applies?

A. ASTM F88
B. ISO 11135
C. ISO 10993
D. ISO 14644

Q627. A 3D-printed titanium implant shows variation in lattice geometry. What must be done?

A. CT scan
B. Hardness test
C. Paint check
D. Label review

Q628. A cloud-linked device sends patient ECGs to physicians. Which safeguard ensures confidentiality?
A. Data encryption
B. Color filter
C. Font update
D. Icon change
Q629. A company replaces its EtO sterilizer control board. What must be redone before release?
A. Training memo
B. Routine audit
C. Label review
D. Requalification test
Q630. What ensures AI diagnostic software remains accurate after model updates?
A. Re-validation plan
B. New logo design
C. Sales training
D. Color change
Q631. A validation engineer tests automated vision inspection for syringes. What parameter defines success?
A. Detection rate
B. Light color
C. Noise level
D. Label font
Q632. Which method confirms bioburden reduction before sterilization?
A. Pre-sterilization count
B. Post-sterilization scan
C. Label inspection
D. Box strength test
Q633. A hospital validates reprocessing of robotic instruments. What evidence is critical?
A. Purchase record
B. User training file
C. Shift schedule list
D. Residual protein data
Q634. Which control maintains stable temperature in cold-chain device manufacturing?
A. Environmental monitoring
B. Label update
C. Batch note
D. Visual audit
Q635. A supplier offers pre-validated sterilization services. What must auditors verify?
A. Validation records
B. Delivery speed
C. Price agreement
D. Label style
Q636. Engineers introduce laser welding for plastic housings. What validation confirms weld integrity?
A. Tensile strength test
B. Color test
C. Odor check
D. Paint thickness
Q637. A mobile-health app processes ECG data. Which standard applies?

A. IEC 62304
B. ISO 10993
C. ISO 11137
D. ISO 14644

Q638. A risk-management review detects new hazard sources after software update. What must occur?

A. Sales training
B. Marketing review
C. Label design
D. Risk file update

Q639. A production line adds automated torque sensors. What study ensures reliability?

A. Calibration study
B. Color test
C. Label check
D. Audit note

Q640. A device uses biodegradable polymers for implants. What testing validates degradation behavior?

A. In-vitro degradation study
B. Label inspection
C. Shipping test
D. Color analysis

Q641. A facility upgrades its sterilizer software to an AI-based control system. What must be proven before use?

A. Staff survey
B. Label redesign
C. Manual update
D. Software validation

Q642. Engineers replace the metal housing of a defibrillator with composite plastic. What must be demonstrated?

A. Electrical shielding
B. Paint adhesion
C. Label clarity
D. Box dimension

Q643. A 3-D printed implant manufacturer modifies powder recycling limits. What validation is required?

A. Material qualification
B. Label audit
C. Cost review
D. Logo test

Q644. A firm adds Bluetooth telemetry to cardiac monitors. What new risk must be assessed?

A. Data interception
B. Color mismatch
C. Box durability
D. Label adhesive

Q645. Validation of a sterile barrier system shows seal strength below limits. What action ensures compliance?

A. Extend label text
B. Hold shipment only

C. Change ink color
D. Re-seal and re-validate

Q646. A risk-management review finds a new hazard in design software. What must engineers do?
A. Update risk file
B. Ignore finding
C. Delay production
D. Send memo

Q647. A sterilization run is interrupted mid-cycle. What is the correct response?
A. Reprocess load
B. Ship anyway
C. Record note
D. Change label

Q648. A new sensor monitors bioburden automatically. What validation verifies reliability?
A. Correlation study
B. Routine audit
C. Batch label check
D. Operator survey

Q649. Which test demonstrates electrical safety under fault conditions?
A. Paint durability
B. Label readability
C. Color uniformity
D. Dielectric strength

Q650. A company switches to biodegradable device packaging. Which validation confirms functionality?
A. Shelf-life study
B. Label inspection
C. Price analysis
D. Color test

Q651. A robotic assembly line shows inconsistent torque values. What analysis should be performed?
A. GR&R study
B. Logo audit
C. Label proof
D. Cost report

Q652. A reprocessing validation fails to remove detergent residues. What must be changed?
A. Rinse cycle
B. Label color
C. Operator note
D. Box design

Q653. A company implements blockchain for device traceability. What evidence confirms valid use?
A. Photo catalog
B. Label sample
C. Font test
D. Immutable records

Q654. A new laser etching machine marks UDI codes. What must be verified?
A. Code readability
B. Laser color
C. Box weight
D. Font size

Q655. A biocompatibility study detects extractables beyond limits. What should be done?
A. Change material
B. Keep as is
C. Delay audit
D. File note
Q656. Which process verifies that sterilization equipment installation meets specifications?
A. Installation qualification
B. Performance qualification
C. Operational qualification
D. Design qualification
Q657. A software bug causes wrong dose calculation in an infusion pump. What must occur?
A. Sales pause
B. Label redesign
C. Operator memo
D. CAPA and re-validation
Q658. A device requires uniform radiation dose distribution. Which validation ensures this?
A. Dosimetry mapping
B. Label print test
C. Box drop test
D. Weight check
Q659. A smart device tracks body temperature and uploads data. What must validation confirm?
A. Accuracy and encryption
B. Label color balance
C. Shelf design review
D. Logo placement
Q660. A device's software upgrade adds machine-learning diagnostics. What testing verifies accuracy?
A. Sales data audit
B. Label layout check
C. Training count review
D. Clinical performance validation
Q661. A manufacturer adds a UV-C disinfection feature to its ventilators. What validation must be performed first?
A. Microbial efficacy
B. Power rating
C. Color uniformity
D. Label layout
Q662. A team replaces a metal catheter connector with polymer. Which test confirms mechanical safety?
A. Tensile strength
B. Color stability
C. Font spacing
D. Box weight
Q663. A company implements predictive-maintenance sensors on sterilizers. What must validation demonstrate?
A. Data accuracy
B. Label color
C. Noise limit
D. Logo size

Q664. An AI tool classifies X-ray images for fracture detection. Which evaluation ensures model fairness?

A. Cost sheet

B. Label check

C. Server log

D. Demographic testing

Q665. A biocompatibility audit finds missing extractable-profile data. What corrective action is required?

A. Conduct testing

B. Delay audit

C. Add note

D. Update logo

Q666. A cleanroom alarm reports differential-pressure loss. What should staff do immediately?

A. Stop production

B. Adjust labels

C. Note incident

D. Repaint walls

Q667. A device's software now connects to external hospital servers. What added risk needs validation?

A. Network security

B. Text contrast

C. Carton design

D. Font style

Q668. A company introduces AI-driven visual inspection. Which measure proves effectiveness?

A. Label size

B. Power usage

C. Paint tone

D. Detection rate

Q669. Engineers add vibration monitoring for packaging lines. What analysis verifies stability?

A. Frequency response

B. Label audit

C. Color chart

D. Weight record

Q670. A new polymer catheter coating reduces friction. Which property must be validated?

A. Lubricity retention

B. Label font

C. Tube color

D. Box finish

Q671. A start-up uses additive manufacturing for bone scaffolds. What critical test ensures porosity design meets spec?

A. Micro-CT analysis

B. Tensile check

C. Label print

D. Carton drop

Q672. Validation of a mobile app interface finds small text unreadable by seniors. What correction aligns with usability standards?

A. Extend label

B. Add symbol

C. Change color
D. Increase font
Q673. An automated washer records cycle parameters electronically. What ensures records remain tamper-proof?
A. Audit trail
B. Label barcode
C. Shift log
D. Cost note
Q674. Engineers qualify a new EtO sterilizer chamber. Which step comes first?
A. Installation qualification
B. Performance qualification
C. Operational qualification
D. Design qualification
Q675. A wearable ECG patch integrates wireless charging. What hazard must risk management include?
A. Thermal injury
B. Label fading
C. Strap color
D. Box size
Q676. A supplier changes sterilant gas purity level. What must be demonstrated?
A. Cost update
B. Label revision
C. Invoice review
D. Process equivalence
Q677. A developer introduces AI-based defect prediction. What ongoing control maintains reliability?
A. Model monitoring
B. Label change
C. User survey
D. Cost audit
Q678. A production robot is relocated to a new room. What must be done first?
A. Re-qualification
B. Label inspection
C. Paint check
D. Staff notice
Q679. A designer evaluates a new anti-fog coating on surgical lenses. Which test verifies clarity?
A. Optical transmittance
B. Color grading
C. Box impact
D. Label density
Q680. A firm adopts cloud-based QMS software. What control ensures data authenticity?
A. Icon color
B. Font template
C. File name
D. Access management
Q681. A validation team verifies robotic-arm calibration for implant assembly. What parameter must meet specification?
A. Positional accuracy
B. Color brightness

C. Label border
D. Carton layout

Q682. A software-controlled autoclave fails to reach target pressure mid-cycle. What is the immediate required action?

A. Abort cycle
B. Adjust timer
C. Update label
D. Record note

Q683. An additive-manufactured bone scaffold exhibits inconsistent pore size. Which test confirms conformity?

A. 3D scan
B. Drop test
C. Box lift
D. Font check

Q684. A medical imaging firm upgrades its AI to include real-time lesion detection. What must validation confirm?

A. Font height
B. Screen color
C. Text contrast
D. Accuracy metrics

Q685. A manufacturer transitions from glass to polymer syringes. What mechanical validation ensures safe use?

A. Burst pressure
B. Label tone
C. Cap color
D. Box print

Q686. A supplier introduces a new sterilant gas mix. What must auditors verify before approval?

A. Validation data
B. Label proofs
C. Color samples
D. Storage log

Q687. Engineers discover data transmission errors in a wearable glucose monitor. What must be re-validated?

A. Wireless communication
B. Battery lifespan
C. Strap material
D. Logo placement

Q688. A packaging process consistently fails peel-strength limits. What adjustment resolves this issue?

A. Font spacing
B. Box graphics
C. Tape label
D. Seal parameters

Q689. A risk analysis identifies residual probability of electrical shock. What must the manufacturer document?

A. Benefit–risk justification
B. Color specification
C. Training list
D. Price quote

Q690. A sterilizer's new IoT dashboard monitors pressure remotely. What must validation confirm?
A. Data accuracy
B. Display contrast
C. Font position
D. Icon color
Q691. Which quality tool best identifies potential causes of a recurring manufacturing defect?
A. Histogram
B. Fishbone diagram
C. Pareto chart
D. Control chart
Q692. The primary purpose of a control chart in process monitoring is to:
A. Detect shifts or trends indicating loss of control
B. Compare operator performance
C. Estimate process capability indices
D. Display customer complaints by category
Q693. Which statistical concept defines the probability of rejecting a good lot during sampling inspection?
A. Producer's risk
B. Consumer's risk
C. Type II error
D. Power of a test
Q694. Which of the following is most appropriate when ranking problem categories by cumulative frequency?
A. Scatter diagram
B. Pareto analysis
C. Histogram
D. Control plan
Q695. What does a process capability index (Cpk) of 1.0 indicate?
A. Process mean is centered and stable
B. Process spread equals tolerance width
C. Process spread fits twice within specification limits
D. Process cannot meet requirements
Q696. Which graphical method displays relationships between two quantitative variables?
A. Scatter diagram
B. Run chart
C. Histogram
D. Box plot
Q697. What is the primary objective of Design of Experiments (DOE) in quality improvement?
A. Monitor process stability
B. Identify factors influencing performance
C. Create control limits
D. Plot sample distributions
Q698. A team collects nonconformance counts over time to identify cyclical variation. Which chart is most suitable?
A. Histogram
B. Run chart
C. Pareto chart
D. Matrix diagram

Q699. Failure Mode and Effects Analysis (FMEA) prioritizes risks by evaluating:

A. Severity, occurrence, and detection
B. Frequency and duration
C. Cost and time
D. Likelihood and confidence

Q700. Which data type is measured on a continuous scale?

A. Attribute
B. Discrete
C. Variable
D. Nominal

Answer key and Explanation (601-700)

Q601. Answer: D

Explanation: Software verification confirms algorithms trigger accurate pressure changes under defined input conditions, ensuring process consistency per IEC 62304. Functional or simulated tests only assess outputs, not code logic or validation integrity. SubChapter: Software Validation

Q602. Answer: A

Explanation: Build orientation affects structural strength; mechanical testing validates mechanical equivalence across orientations per ISO/ASTM 52920. Thermal, porosity, and powder-flow tests measure contributing parameters but not overall mechanical consistency. SubChapter: Additive Manufacturing Validation

Q603. Answer: A

Explanation: Unsecured network ports create high vulnerability; implementing patches and verifying through penetration testing mitigates risk under IEC 81001-5-1. Other actions are temporary and fail to address systemic threats. SubChapter: Cybersecurity Risk Management

Q604. Answer: A

Explanation: ISO 14971 defines the framework for identifying, evaluating, controlling, and monitoring risks throughout the product lifecycle. Other standards address sterilization, cleanrooms, and biocompatibility, not comprehensive risk integration. SubChapter: Risk Management Principles

Q605. Answer: C

Explanation: Validating encrypted data transmission and secure access aligns with FDA cybersecurity expectations, ensuring confidentiality and integrity of patient information. Cosmetic or administrative actions cannot secure data flows effectively. SubChapter: Digital Health Security

Q606. Answer: A

Explanation: Heat penetration testing confirms uniform thermal exposure within sterilization loads, validating placement and cycle effectiveness per ISO 17665. Pressure, humidity, or label tests measure unrelated parameters. SubChapter: Sterilization Process Qualification

Q607. Answer: A

Explanation: Redesigning interface layout eliminates use error at the design stage per IEC 62366-1. Labels or training reduce but do not remove human-factor hazards, and brightness adjustments are ineffective. SubChapter: Human Factors Engineering

Q608. Answer: A

Explanation: Gauge Repeatability and Reproducibility quantifies measurement system variation across instruments and users, ensuring reliability of quality data. Other tools identify risks or trends but not measurement precision. SubChapter: Metrology and Process Control

Q609. Answer: D

Explanation: Calibration validation ensures sensors and actuators align within precision limits per IEC 80601-2-77, preventing unsafe motion errors. Interface, power, or cabling rarely resolve positional inaccuracy directly. SubChapter: Robotic Systems Validation

Q610. Answer: A

Explanation: Change request logs formally document engineering changes, justifications, and approvals, ensuring traceability per 21 CFR 820.30(i). Reviews and maintenance logs don't substitute validated change documentation. SubChapter: Design Change Control

Q611. Answer: A

Explanation: Adjusting and re-validating cleaning parameters ensures residue removal meets acceptance limits. ISO 17664 and FDA guidance mandate quantitative control, whereas ignoring or unrelated actions breach safety compliance. SubChapter: Reprocessing Validation

Q612. Answer: A

Explanation: Density mapping identifies voids and ensures solidification quality within additive-manufactured parts. Fatigue or electrical tests evaluate performance but not porosity formation. SubChapter: Additive Manufacturing Quality Control

Q613. Answer: D

Explanation: IEC 60601 governs safety and essential performance requirements for medical electrical equipment worldwide. Other standards address quality, sterilization, and management systems, not electrical safety. SubChapter: Electrical Safety

Q614. Answer: A

Explanation: Routine dose audits confirm sterilization process maintains adequate lethality per ISO 11137-2, safeguarding sterility assurance levels. Other activities don't verify microbial control consistency. SubChapter: Sterilization Validation Maintenance

Q615. Answer: A

Explanation: Particle counting provides quantitative assessment of airborne contamination levels, ensuring compliance with ISO 14644-1 classification. Other methods lack measurable particulate detection. SubChapter: Controlled Environment Monitoring

Q616. Answer: A

Explanation: ISO 14971 and FDA cybersecurity guidance require documented justification showing benefits outweigh residual cybersecurity risks after mitigation. Ignoring or halting without assessment is noncompliant. SubChapter: Cybersecurity Risk Assessment

Q617. Answer: D

Explanation: Calibration verification ensures sensors meet precision specifications critical for environmental qualification. Skill, labeling, or audit status don't ensure measurement integrity. SubChapter: Equipment Qualification

Q618. Answer: A

Explanation: Comparative performance validation between reprocessed and new catheters demonstrates mechanical and functional equivalence, ensuring patient safety compliance with FDA and ISO 17664. Documentation-only measures don't verify equivalence. SubChapter: Reprocessing Validation

Q619. Answer: A

Explanation: Algorithm validation ensures consistent diagnostic accuracy across datasets and demographics, preventing bias or misclassification per GMLP. Labeling or physical attributes are unrelated to software performance. SubChapter: AI Validation

Q620. Answer: A

Explanation: Installation Qualification confirms utilities and equipment conform to design and specification requirements before operational testing. PQ and OQ validate later performance; DQ defines conceptual needs. SubChapter: Equipment Qualification

Q621. Answer: D

Explanation: Regular chamber calibration confirms sensors maintain accuracy within validated limits, ensuring consistent sterilization performance per ISO 17665. Notes or labels don't verify measurement accuracy, and shipment delays without correction leave risk unresolved. SubChapter: Sterilization Process Control

Q622. Answer: A

Explanation: Wear testing under simulated physiological conditions quantifies durability and friction coefficient stability, verifying coating performance per ASTM F732. Visual or documentation checks can't confirm functional integrity. SubChapter: Surface Engineering Validation

Q623. Answer: A

Explanation: Detection-accuracy validation ensures robots reliably identify defects within tolerance limits, maintaining product conformity. IEC 80601-2-77 and ISO 9283 emphasize precision and repeatability. Speed or aesthetics don't assure detection reliability. SubChapter: Automation Validation

Q624. Answer: A
Explanation: Any material-formulation change requires repeat ISO 10993 biocompatibility testing to confirm absence of cytotoxic or sensitization effects. Administrative reviews don't confirm biological safety, and waivers violate regulatory control. SubChapter: Material Change Validation
Q625. Answer: D
Explanation: Connectivity testing validates reliable, secure data transfer between inhaler and mobile app per FDA digital-health guidance. Cosmetic or logistical checks don't guarantee accurate communication. SubChapter: Connected Device Verification
Q626. Answer: A
Explanation: ASTM F88 measures seal tensile strength, confirming package integrity under handling stress. ISO 11135 covers EtO sterilization, ISO 10993 biocompatibility, and ISO 14644 cleanroom standards. SubChapter: Packaging Validation
Q627. Answer: A
Explanation: Computed-tomography scanning verifies internal lattice consistency and detects structural deviations without destruction, meeting ISO/ASTM 52920 quality requirements. Surface or label checks don't reveal internal flaws. SubChapter: Additive Manufacturing Inspection
Q628. Answer: A
Explanation: End-to-end encryption validated under IEC 81001-5-1 maintains data privacy and integrity during transfer. Cosmetic or interface changes offer no security protection, risking HIPAA noncompliance. SubChapter: Cybersecurity and Data Protection
Q629. Answer: D
Explanation: Hardware replacement demands installation and operational requalification to confirm control accuracy per ISO 11135. Administrative reviews alone can't verify equipment reliability or sterility assurance. SubChapter: Equipment Requalification
Q630. Answer: A
Explanation: A documented re-validation plan verifies updated AI models maintain performance metrics and bias controls, satisfying FDA GMLP expectations. Visual or marketing changes don't confirm algorithmic reliability. SubChapter: AI/ML Lifecycle Validation
Q631. Answer: A
Explanation: Detection-rate validation quantifies system sensitivity and specificity in defect identification, demonstrating process effectiveness. Environmental or aesthetic factors don't measure detection performance. SubChapter: Automation Process Validation
Q632. Answer: A
Explanation: Measuring bioburden before sterilization establishes baseline microbial load, essential for dose setting under ISO 11737-1. Post-sterilization or packaging checks cannot characterize initial contamination. SubChapter: Microbiological Testing
Q633. Answer: D
Explanation: Residual-protein assay confirms cleaning efficacy and material compatibility after repeated cycles, per ISO 17664 and FDA guidance. Administrative or procurement documents provide no proof of cleanliness. SubChapter: Reprocessing Validation
Q634. Answer: A
Explanation: Continuous environmental monitoring ensures temperature and humidity remain within validated limits, preventing degradation of sensitive materials. Documentation changes don't maintain physical conditions. SubChapter: Controlled Environment Management
Q635. Answer: A
Explanation: Reviewing sterilization validation evidence ensures compliance with ISO 11137 or 11135 and confirms microbial lethality. Non-technical factors like pricing or labels don't prove process adequacy. SubChapter: Supplier Validation

Q636. Answer: A
Explanation: Tensile testing verifies weld joint strength and consistency under mechanical stress, ensuring reliable bonding in production. Surface or sensory tests provide no mechanical assurance. SubChapter: Process Validation
Q637. Answer: A
Explanation: IEC 62304 specifies lifecycle software development and maintenance requirements for safety-critical medical apps. Biocompatibility, sterilization, or cleanroom standards are unrelated. SubChapter: Software Lifecycle Management
Q638. Answer: D
Explanation: ISO 14971 requires immediate risk-file updates and re-evaluation when new hazards appear to ensure continuous safety compliance. Non-technical reviews cannot control emerging risks. SubChapter: Risk Management Maintenance
Q639. Answer: A
Explanation: Calibration studies confirm sensors measure within specified tolerances under load, validating torque control accuracy. Cosmetic or paperwork changes provide no measurement verification. SubChapter: Metrology and Automation
Q640. Answer: A
Explanation: Controlled in-vitro degradation testing simulates physiological conditions to confirm predictable mass loss and mechanical performance over time, meeting ISO 10993-13 guidance. Surface or shipping checks lack mechanistic data. SubChapter: Biodegradable Material Validation
Q641. Answer: D
Explanation: Validating AI control algorithms ensures temperature and pressure remain within sterilization limits, maintaining sterility assurance per IEC 62304 and ISO 11135. Administrative or aesthetic updates offer no evidence of process control or safety performance. SubChapter: Software-Integrated Sterilization
Q642. Answer: A
Explanation: Electrical-shielding verification confirms the new composite provides equivalent electromagnetic protection per IEC 60601-1-2. Surface or visual inspections cannot prove EMC compliance or device safety under field conditions. SubChapter: Electromagnetic Compatibility
Q643. Answer: A
Explanation: Material qualification testing confirms recycled powder retains mechanical, chemical, and biocompatibility properties, ensuring part equivalence per ISO/ASTM 52907. Administrative or branding activities don't verify powder integrity or consistency. SubChapter: Additive Manufacturing Material Control
Q644. Answer: A
Explanation: Wireless connectivity introduces cybersecurity and privacy threats; risk analysis must address data interception per FDA cybersecurity guidance and IEC 81001-5-1. Cosmetic or packaging issues do not affect information security. SubChapter: Cybersecurity Risk Assessment
Q645. Answer: D
Explanation: Re-sealing with adjusted temperature, pressure, or dwell time followed by validation under ASTM F88 confirms packaging integrity. Holding shipments or cosmetic changes don't correct seal deficiencies or restore compliance. SubChapter: Packaging Validation
Q646. Answer: A
Explanation: ISO 14971 requires updating the risk management file to capture new hazards and reassess controls. Ignoring or delaying without review creates traceability gaps and regulatory non-conformance. SubChapter: Risk File Maintenance
Q647. Answer: A

Explanation: Interruption compromises sterility assurance; entire load must be reprocessed after equipment requalification to maintain validated conditions under ISO 11135 or 11137. Partial documentation or cosmetic actions don't restore sterility. SubChapter: Sterilization Process Control

Q648. Answer: A

Explanation: Correlation studies compare automated sensor results with standard culture methods to confirm accuracy and linearity per ISO 11737-1. Audits or documentation reviews can't quantify measurement validity. SubChapter: Microbiological Automation Validation

Q649. Answer: D

Explanation: Dielectric-strength testing ensures insulation withstands applied voltage without breakdown, a critical IEC 60601-1 requirement. Aesthetic or surface checks don't evaluate user protection against electric shock. SubChapter: Electrical Safety Testing

Q650. Answer: A

Explanation: Accelerated and real-time shelf-life studies demonstrate barrier stability and mechanical integrity over storage periods per ISO 11607. Cosmetic or financial reviews cannot assure functional performance. SubChapter: Packaging Performance Validation

Q651. Answer: A

Explanation: Gauge Repeatability and Reproducibility studies identify variation from equipment and operators, helping correct torque measurement errors per ISO 22514. Administrative tasks don't measure precision or process capability. SubChapter: Process Control Validation

Q652. Answer: A

Explanation: Adjusting and re-validating rinse cycles ensures residue reduction below toxic limits per ISO 17664. Cosmetic or paperwork changes don't improve cleaning efficacy or compliance. SubChapter: Reprocessing Validation

Q653. Answer: D

Explanation: Verification of immutable, auditable records and controlled access ensures blockchain meets QMS traceability requirements under 21 CFR 820.180. Visual or aesthetic proof offers no data integrity assurance. SubChapter: Digital Traceability Validation

Q654. Answer: A

Explanation: Code-readability testing ensures UDI marks remain legible throughout sterilization and life cycle per ISO 15459 and FDA UDI rules. Cosmetic parameters don't verify identification functionality. SubChapter: Labeling and UDI

Q655. Answer: A

Explanation: Exceeding chemical limits requires material substitution and re-testing to ensure patient safety per ISO 10993-18 and -17. Deferring action or noting only fails regulatory compliance. SubChapter: Biocompatibility Validation

Q656. Answer: A

Explanation: Installation Qualification (IQ) confirms equipment and utilities match design specifications before OQ and PQ testing. Skipping IQ risks invalidating subsequent validation phases. SubChapter: Equipment Qualification

Q657. Answer: D

Explanation: Corrective and Preventive Action followed by software re-validation ensures algorithm accuracy per IEC 62304 and ISO 14971. Administrative steps without testing fail to prove correction effectiveness. SubChapter: Software Risk Control

Q658. Answer: A

Explanation: Dosimetry mapping verifies radiation intensity uniformity throughout the load, ensuring effective sterilization per ISO 11137-1 and -3. Packaging or aesthetic tests cannot assess dose spread. SubChapter: Radiation Sterilization

Q659. Answer: A

Explanation: Validation must demonstrate sensor accuracy and secure data transmission complying with FDA cybersecurity and IEC 81001-5-1. Cosmetic changes don't verify measurement or privacy controls. SubChapter: Digital Health Validation

Q660. Answer: D

Explanation: Clinical performance validation using representative datasets confirms ML diagnostic accuracy and bias control, meeting FDA Good Machine Learning Practice standards. Administrative or marketing checks don't prove safety or effectiveness. SubChapter: AI/ML Performance Validation

Q661. Answer: A

Explanation: Microbial-efficacy testing verifies UV-C intensity achieves required log-reduction of pathogens under real-use conditions, ensuring patient safety. Power or color checks don't confirm germicidal performance, and labeling adds no biological assurance. SubChapter: Alternative Sterilization Technologies**

Q662. Answer: A

Explanation: Tensile-strength testing ensures polymer connectors withstand applied forces equal to or exceeding the original design per ISO 80369. Visual or packaging assessments cannot verify functional safety or connection reliability. SubChapter: Mechanical Integrity Validation**

Q663. Answer: A

Explanation: Predictive-maintenance validation confirms sensor readings accurately detect deviations in pressure or temperature, preventing process drift and downtime. Other variables affect aesthetics only and do not prove data reliability. SubChapter: Smart Equipment Validation**

Q664. Answer: D

Explanation: Demographic performance testing ensures algorithmic equity across age, sex, and ethnicity, aligning with FDA GMLP fairness expectations. Administrative records cannot reveal bias or diagnostic imbalance. SubChapter: AI/ML Fairness Assessment**

Q665. Answer: A

Explanation: Extractables and leachables testing identifies potential chemical migration from device materials per ISO 10993-18, confirming patient safety. Documentation changes alone cannot supply missing toxicological data. SubChapter: Biocompatibility Validation**

Q666. Answer: A

Explanation: Production must halt until positive-pressure balance is restored and verified per ISO 14644-2, preventing contamination migration. Merely noting or cosmetic actions fail to protect product sterility. SubChapter: Controlled Environment Management**

Q667. Answer: A

Explanation: Network-security validation tests encryption, authentication, and data-access control per IEC 81001-5-1, ensuring confidentiality and system integrity. Interface or packaging aspects don't address cybersecurity exposure. SubChapter: Cybersecurity Validation**

Q668. Answer: D

Explanation: Measuring detection rate and false-rejection ratio validates AI inspection accuracy, supporting release decisions under ISO TR 20416 guidelines. Cosmetic or energy data fail to confirm defect-detection capability. SubChapter: Automated Inspection Validation**

Q669. Answer: A

Explanation: Frequency-response analysis identifies resonance that can damage seals or contents, ensuring system stability and compliance with ASTM D4169 transport standards. Administrative checks don't assess vibration behavior. SubChapter: Packaging Process Qualification**

Q670. Answer: A

Explanation: Lubricity-retention validation measures dynamic friction before and after aging or sterilization, confirming sustained performance per ASTM D1894. Appearance changes don't demonstrate coating durability or usability. SubChapter: Surface Performance Testing**

Q671. Answer: A
Explanation: Micro-CT analysis provides 3-D quantitative porosity mapping, verifying structural uniformity essential for osteointegration, per ISO/ASTM 52921. Mechanical or packaging tests can't characterize internal geometry. SubChapter: Additive Manufacturing Quality**
Q672. Answer: D
Explanation: Increasing font size and contrast enhances accessibility and meets IEC 62366-1 usability design principles. Symbols or color shifts may not address readability for target demographics. SubChapter: Human Factors Engineering**
Q673. Answer: A
Explanation: Secure audit trails protect data integrity and traceability per 21 CFR Part 11 and ISO 13485 § 4.2.5, verifying authenticity of electronic cleaning records. Non-controlled logs are insufficient. SubChapter: Electronic Record Validation**
Q674. Answer: A
Explanation: Installation Qualification confirms proper setup, utilities, and instrumentation before OQ and PQ begin, ensuring baseline accuracy per ISO 11135. Later phases rely on verified installation results. SubChapter: Equipment Qualification**
Q675. Answer: A
Explanation: Wireless charging introduces potential surface heating; evaluating skin-temperature rise prevents burns, complying with ISO 14971 risk-control requirements. Cosmetic issues pose no patient hazard. SubChapter: Risk Assessment for Emerging Tech**
Q676. Answer: D
Explanation: Process-equivalence validation ensures altered gas composition maintains microbial lethality and material compatibility per ISO 11135. Documentation updates alone don't confirm sterilization consistency. SubChapter: Sterilization Process Validation**
Q677. Answer: A
Explanation: Continuous model-monitoring tracks accuracy drift and triggers retraining when prediction error rises, sustaining validated performance per FDA adaptive-AI guidance. Non-technical reviews can't ensure predictive integrity. SubChapter: AI/ML Maintenance**
Q678. Answer: A
Explanation: Environmental changes affect alignment and calibration; full re-qualification verifies repeatability, safety interlocks, and precision per ISO 10218. Administrative actions alone don't re-establish validated status. SubChapter: Equipment Re-qualification**
Q679. Answer: A
Explanation: Measuring optical transmittance before and after exposure quantifies coating performance under humidity, ensuring visibility compliance with ISO 10993-1 and ASTM D1003. Cosmetic or packaging assessments don't verify clarity retention. SubChapter: Surface Property Validation**
Q680. Answer: D
Explanation: Controlled user authentication and permission layers protect data authenticity and traceability per 21 CFR Part 11 and ISO 13485 electronic-record requirements. Visual formatting has no effect on security or validation integrity. SubChapter: Digital QMS Compliance**
Q681. Answer: A
Explanation: Positional-accuracy verification ensures robotic movements stay within micrometer tolerances required for precision assembly, maintaining patient safety and ISO 9283 compliance. Visual or packaging attributes provide no evidence of mechanical accuracy or functional precision. SubChapter: Robotic System Validation**
Q682. Answer: A

Explanation: Aborting the cycle prevents incomplete sterilization and protects product sterility assurance. ISO 17665 requires reprocessing of affected loads after correction. Timing or documentation updates do not eliminate sterility failure risk. SubChapter: Sterilization Process Control**

Q683. Answer: A

Explanation: High-resolution 3D scanning quantifies pore geometry and uniformity, confirming scaffold structure meets design and mechanical criteria per ISO/ASTM 52921. Physical handling or visual checks cannot detect internal pore irregularities. SubChapter: Additive Manufacturing Verification**

Q684. Answer: D

Explanation: Validation must verify AI output accuracy, sensitivity, and specificity using representative clinical data per FDA Good Machine Learning Practice. Interface or visual changes don't evaluate algorithm performance or diagnostic safety. SubChapter: AI Diagnostic Validation**

Q685. Answer: A

Explanation: Burst-pressure testing evaluates syringe wall strength and sealing integrity, ensuring polymer durability under use pressures per ISO 7886-1. Aesthetic or labeling inspections don't measure containment performance or patient safety. SubChapter: Material Substitution Validation**

Q686. Answer: A

Explanation: Reviewing sterilization validation data confirms microbial lethality, material compatibility, and regulatory compliance per ISO 11135. Non-technical documentation cannot verify process effectiveness or product safety. SubChapter: Supplier Process Validation**

Q687. Answer: A

Explanation: Wireless validation ensures data packets transmit accurately and securely between device and application per IEC 60601-1-2 and FDA guidance. Physical design elements cannot fix or verify communication integrity. SubChapter: Connected Device Validation**

Q688. Answer: D

Explanation: Adjusting sealing temperature, pressure, and dwell time followed by re-validation under ASTM F88 re-establishes packaging integrity. Aesthetic or labeling modifications cannot correct structural sealing performance. SubChapter: Packaging Process Validation**

Q689. Answer: A

Explanation: ISO 14971 requires documented benefit–risk justification when residual risk remains after controls, ensuring transparency in acceptance rationale. Administrative or commercial details have no bearing on safety evaluation. SubChapter: Residual Risk Documentation**

Q690. Answer: A

Explanation: Validation must demonstrate transmitted data accuracy and synchronization with system readings, ensuring integrity under ISO 17665 and IEC 81001-5-1. Interface cosmetics do not affect reliability of monitoring or record accuracy. SubChapter: IoT-Enabled Sterilization Validation**

Q691. Answer: B

Explanation: The fishbone diagram organizes possible defect causes into structured categories. Option A – Shows distribution, not causation. Option C – Ranks frequency, not relationships. Option D – Monitors variation, not root causes.

Chapter V – Quality Tools & Techniques

Q692. Answer: A

Explanation: Control charts reveal instability through trend or limit violations. Option B – Focuses on personnel, not process. Option C – Requires separate capability study. Option D – Represents a Pareto, not SPC, function.

Chapter V – Quality Tools & Techniques

Q693. Answer: A

Explanation: Producer's risk (α) is rejecting a conforming lot. Option B – Consumer's risk accepts bad lots. Option C – Applies to hypothesis tests. Option D – Inverse of Type II error.

Chapter V – Quality Tools & Techniques
Q694. Answer: B
Explanation: Pareto analysis orders problems by frequency to focus on the vital few. Option A – Shows correlation. Option C – Shows distribution only. Option D – Defines control actions, not ranking.
Chapter V – Quality Tools & Techniques
Q695. Answer: B
Explanation: Cpk = 1.0 means process variation equals tolerance; about 99.73 % within limits. Option A – Centering affects Cp vs Cpk. Option C – Overstates capability. Option D – Incorrect; it meets limits.
Chapter V – Quality Tools & Techniques
Q696. Answer: A
Explanation: Scatter diagrams visualize variable correlation. Option B – Tracks time-based trends. Option C – Shows one-variable distribution. Option D – Summarizes spread, not correlation.
Chapter V – Quality Tools & Techniques
Q697. Answer: B
Explanation: DOE determines key variables affecting outcomes. Option A – SPC task. Option C – Derived from data, not DOE. Option D – Descriptive only.
Chapter V – Quality Tools & Techniques
Q698. Answer: B
Explanation: Run charts reveal time-based patterns and cycles. Option A – Shows distribution, not sequence. Option C – Ranks categories. Option D – Maps relationships, not time.
Chapter V – Quality Tools & Techniques
Q699. Answer: A
Explanation: FMEA uses severity, occurrence, and detection to compute RPN. Option B – Incomplete. Option C – Business not safety. Option D – Generic risk terms.
Chapter V – Quality Tools & Techniques
Q700. Answer: C
Explanation: Variable data are measurable and continuous (e.g., length, weight). Option A – Pass/fail. Option B – Count-based. Option D – Categorical.
Chapter V – Quality Tools & Techniques

Questions (701-800)

Q701. The main reason to construct a cause-and-effect matrix is to:

A. Display control chart data
B. Link process inputs to customer outputs
C. Rank inspection results
D. Record supplier performance

Q702. What is the primary function of benchmarking in quality management?

A. Establish process control limits
B. Compare performance against best practices
C. Quantify defect severity
D. Analyze failure modes

Q703. Which tool best displays interactions between multiple process variables in a designed experiment?

A. Interaction plot
B. Histogram
C. Pareto chart
D. Flowchart

Q704. When a control chart shows seven consecutive points on one side of the mean, it signals:

A. Random variation
B. Special cause variation
C. Stable process
D. Sampling error

Q705. Which risk-management tool supports prioritization of hazards in device design?

A. Fault Tree Analysis
B. SIPOC diagram
C. Check sheet
D. Histogram

Q706. What statistical test is most suitable to compare means of more than two groups?

A. t-test
B. ANOVA
C. Chi-square test
D. F-test for variance

Q707. Which method helps determine whether observed variation is due to measurement system error?

A. Gauge R&R study
B. Control chart
C. Capability analysis
D. Regression

Q708. What tool best displays cumulative contribution of categories toward a total?

A. Histogram
B. Pareto chart
C. Check sheet
D. Scatter diagram

Q709. The 5 Whys technique primarily assists in:

A. Establishing control limits
B. Root cause identification
C. Data classification

D. Risk prioritization

Q710. Which analytical tool quantifies potential benefits of improvement alternatives using probability and impact?

A. Decision tree analysis
B. Histogram
C. Control chart
D. Affinity diagram

Q711. Which graphical tool best helps identify whether measurement errors come from repeatability or reproducibility issues?

A. Histogram
B. Scatter diagram
C. Gauge R&R study
D. Control chart

Q712. Which tool assists a team in systematically arranging ideas into logical categories during brainstorming?

A. Affinity diagram
B. Pareto chart
C. Flowchart
D. Histogram

Q713. Which analytical method determines how multiple input factors collectively influence a single output?

A. ANOVA
B. DOE
C. Regression analysis
D. Control plan

Q714. Which quality planning tool is used to visualize project tasks, timelines, and dependencies?

A. Gantt chart
B. Flowchart
C. Scatter plot
D. Pareto diagram

Q715. Which statistical measure reflects the central tendency of a normally distributed dataset?

A. Range
B. Median
C. Mean
D. Mode

Q716. What is the main benefit of using control charts for continuous process monitoring?

A. Detects nonrandom variation early
B. Measures operator efficiency
C. Calculates specification limits
D. Documents inspection frequency

Q717. Which tool would an auditor use to identify the step in a process where a defect most likely occurs?

A. Flowchart
B. Control plan
C. Run chart
D. Histogram

Q718. Which risk assessment tool visually decomposes events leading to a system failure?

A. Fishbone diagram

B. Fault Tree Analysis
C. Pareto chart
D. Scatter diagram
Q719. What is the purpose of process capability analysis?
A. Determine if a process can meet specifications
B. Identify out-of-control signals
C. Measure operator performance
D. Evaluate data normality
Q720. Which diagram is best suited for showing a process and associated decision points?
A. Flowchart
B. Histogram
C. Control chart
D. Matrix diagram
Q721. Which quality improvement tool ranks problems by weighted importance based on team consensus?
A. Prioritization matrix
B. Check sheet
C. Histogram
D. Scatter plot
Q722. Which tool supports decision-making by comparing potential outcomes and associated probabilities?
A. Control chart
B. Flowchart
C. Pareto chart
D. Decision tree
Q723. In process analysis, what is the main purpose of a scatter diagram?
A. Identify correlation between variables
B. Monitor stability over time
C. Rank causes by impact
D. Display categorical proportions
Q724. Which technique helps a team understand process variability and its sources before implementing controls?
A. Cause-and-effect diagram
B. Control chart
C. Check sheet
D. Pareto chart
Q725. Which statistical term quantifies the proportion of total variation explained by a regression model?
A. R^2 coefficient
B. p-value
C. Standard error
D. Mean square
Q726. What type of data would result from counting the number of defective units in a lot?
A. Variable
B. Attribute
C. Nominal
D. Ordinal
Q727. Which visualization displays how often different values occur within a data set?

A. Histogram
B. Control chart
C. Pareto diagram
D. Scatter plot

Q728. Which advanced analysis helps determine whether observed process variation stems from random error or assignable causes?
A. Statistical Process Control (SPC)
B. Design of Experiments
C. Reliability analysis
D. Benchmarking

Q729. What is the key objective of using a check sheet in data collection?
A. Ensure data are collected consistently at the source
B. Rank root causes
C. Estimate population mean
D. Detect out-of-control signals

Q730. Which visual management tool summarizes project progress through color-coded task status indicators?
A. Dashboard
B. Histogram
C. Scatter plot
D. Control chart

Q731. Which method determines whether process variation comes mainly from machines, operators, or materials?
A. Design of Experiments
B. Gauge R&R study
C. ANOVA
D. Regression analysis

Q732. Which diagram clarifies the logical sequence and interdependencies of process activities?
A. Flowchart
B. Pareto chart
C. Fishbone diagram
D. Histogram

Q733. Which improvement tool visually identifies the largest contributors to a quality issue?
A. Pareto chart
B. Control chart
C. Scatter diagram
D. Affinity diagram

Q734. What is the main objective of a cause-and-Correct Answer: effect diagram?
A. Display process performance over time
B. Identify potential root causes of a problem
C. Quantify process capability indices
D. Rank project priorities

Q735. Which statistical tool measures linear correlation strength between two variables?
A. Regression analysis
B. ANOVA
C. Chi-square test
D. Histogram

Q736. Which type of data arises from pass/fail or go/no-go inspection?

A. Attribute
B. Variable
C. Ordinal
D. Interval

Q737. Which chart best detects gradual process drifts before specifications are exceeded?
A. Run chart
B. Control chart
C. Pareto chart
D. Histogram

Q738. What is the purpose of a box-and-whisker plot?
A. Display defect frequencies
B. Show data spread and outliers
C. Depict process steps
D. Rank causes by importance

Q739. Which method ensures balanced data collection across multiple operators and instruments?
A. Gauge R&R design
B. Random sampling
C. Stratified sampling
D. Control plan

Q740. Which quality technique compares performance metrics against recognized industry leaders?
A. Benchmarking
B. DOE
C. SPC
D. FMEA

Q741. Which control-chart pattern indicates over-control or tampering with a stable process?
A. Frequent point oscillation around center line
B. Seven points on one side of mean
C. Sudden jump beyond limits
D. Consistent downward trend

Q742. Which reliability metric measures the probability a device will function for a specified time?
A. Mean Time Between Failures (MTBF)
B. Cpk
C. Sigma level
D. R^2 value

Q743. Which statistical test determines if observed frequencies differ significantly from expected values?
A. ANOVA
B. t-test
C. F-test
D. Chi-square test

Q744. What is the key goal of process mapping?
A. Define inputs and outputs for each activity
B. Measure operator accuracy
C. Estimate process capability
D. Calculate risk priority numbers

Q745. Which measure quantifies how many standard deviations fit between the process mean and nearest specification limit?
A. Cpk

B. Cp
C. Sigma level
D. Z-score

Q746. Which structured brainstorming method encourages equal participation by ranking ideas anonymously?

A. Nominal group technique
B. Affinity diagram
C. Focus group
D. Fishbone analysis

Q747. Which SPC rule signals a possible process shift?

A. Two of three points near a control limit
B. Alternating up-down pattern
C. Isolated point near centerline
D. Five points within $\pm 1\sigma$

Q748. What is the first step in constructing a Pareto chart?

A. Collect frequency data by category
B. Compute process capability indices
C. Establish control limits
D. Develop Ishikawa diagram

Q749. Which reliability analysis graph plots cumulative failure probability over time?

A. Control chart
B. Run chart
C. Histogram
D. Weibull plot

Q750. Which analytical approach combines severity, occurrence, and detection to prioritize corrective actions?

A. FMEA
B. SPC
C. Benchmarking
D. DOE

Q751. Which statistical method evaluates the relationship strength and direction between two continuous variables?

A. Regression analysis
B. ANOVA
C. Chi-square test
D. Control chart

Q752. Which tool identifies and categorizes potential causes contributing to a single effect?

A. Fishbone diagram
B. Pareto chart
C. Histogram
D. Flowchart

Q753. What is the key purpose of a control plan in a quality system?

A. Document methods for sustaining process performance
B. Track project milestones
C. Rank quality problems
D. Evaluate supplier performance

Q754. Which data collection method ensures consistent observation recording during inspections?

A. Control chart

B. Flowchart
C. Pareto chart
D. Check sheet

Q755. What is the principal function of Statistical Process Control (SPC)?
A. Detect special causes of variation
B. Rank failure modes
C. Compare supplier performance
D. Evaluate customer satisfaction

Q756. Which chart type displays how multiple categorical variables relate to one another?
A. Matrix diagram
B. Histogram
C. Run chart
D. Scatter plot

Q757. In FMEA, what does a high Risk Priority Number (RPN) indicate?
A. Greater potential impact and need for corrective action
B. Lower occurrence probability
C. Strong process control
D. Acceptable risk level

Q758. Which tool is most suitable for monitoring defect rates over time for attribute data?
A. p-chart
B. c-chart
C. $\bar{X}$-R chart
D. Run chart

Q759. What is the first step in conducting a root cause analysis?
A. Brainstorm potential causes
B. Implement corrective action immediately
C. Gather measurement data
D. Clearly define the problem statement

Q760. Which improvement methodology uses DMAIC as its structured problem-solving approach?
A. Six Sigma
B. Lean manufacturing
C. ISO 9001
D. Total Quality Management

Q761. Which graphical tool helps identify whether improvement actions reduced process variability?
A. Control chart
B. Pareto diagram
C. Flowchart
D. Check sheet

Q762. Which technique measures process capability for continuous data with known specification limits?
A. Cp and Cpk indices
B. RPN calculation
C. ANOVA
D. F-test

Q763. What is the key benefit of using scatter diagrams during process improvement?
A. Establishes control limits
B. Confirms process stability
C. Defines inspection intervals

D. Reveals possible relationships between variables

Q764. Which Lean tool aims to identify and eliminate non–value-added steps in a process?

A. Value Stream Mapping
B. Pareto analysis
C. ANOVA
D. Cause-and-effect diagram

Q765. Which chart type is best for analyzing defect counts per unit when sample sizes are constant?

A. c-chart
B. p-chart
C. $\bar{X}$ chart
D. Scatter plot

Q766. What is the primary goal of using the 5S methodology in quality improvement?

A. Create organized, efficient, and clean workplaces
B. Identify root causes of variation
C. Measure operator productivity
D. Define design inputs

Q767. Which tool is designed to prioritize potential process changes by comparing expected benefits against required effort?

A. FMEA
B. Control chart
C. Histogram
D. Impact-effort matrix

Q768. What is the function of a run chart in process analysis?

A. Display trends or shifts over time
B. Measure process capability
C. Rank issues by frequency
D. Illustrate cause-and-effect

Q769. Which statistical concept measures how spread out data values are around the mean?

A. Standard deviation
B. Mean
C. Median
D. Range

Q770. Which quality improvement technique involves observing actual work to identify inefficiencies directly?

A. Gemba walk
B. Control chart
C. Pareto analysis
D. Flowcharting

Q771. Which tool helps determine if a measurement process consistently produces the same results under unchanged conditions?

A. Scatter plot
B. Control chart
C. Pareto diagram
D. Repeatability study

Q772. Which tool assists in visualizing multiple possible failure pathways that could lead to a system malfunction?

A. Fault Tree Analysis
B. Histogram

C. Run chart
D. Check sheet

Q773. What is the primary advantage of using a cause-and-effect matrix?
A. Prioritizes process inputs that strongly affect customer outputs
B. Establishes control limits for process variation
C. Defines supplier quality metrics
D. Calculates process capability indices

Q774. Which improvement methodology focuses on reducing process waste and increasing efficiency?
A. Lean
B. Six Sigma
C. FMEA
D. Benchmarking

Q775. What is the main goal of measurement system analysis (MSA)?
A. Identify major process bottlenecks
B. Determine supplier reliability
C. Establish customer satisfaction trends
D. Evaluate accuracy and precision of the measurement process

Q776. Which chart is used for monitoring the number of defects per unit when sample sizes vary?
A. u-chart
B. c-chart
C. p-chart
D. $\bar{X}$-R chart

Q777. Which tool is most effective for visually separating common from special causes of variation?
A. Control chart
B. Histogram
C. Check sheet
D. Pareto chart

Q778. Which analysis technique estimates a device's reliability using time-to-failure data?
A. Weibull analysis
B. DOE
C. ANOVA
D. Benchmarking

Q779. What is the first step when constructing a histogram?
A. Identify root causes
B. Collect and organize continuous data into logical intervals
C. Compute control limits
D. Define failure modes

Q780. Which visual tool compares process performance against target specifications in a single view?
A. Capability histogram
B. Scatter plot
C. Flowchart
D. Check sheet

Q781. What is the key purpose of an Ishikawa diagram in a corrective action team?
A. Brainstorm and categorize possible root causes
B. Track corrective action completion
C. Measure failure probability
D. Compare supplier performance

Q782. Which chart is appropriate for analyzing continuous data where subgroup averages are tracked over time?
A. $\bar{X}$-R chart
B. p-chart
C. c-chart
D. Run chart
Q783. Which quality improvement concept emphasizes prevention of errors through system design?
A. Poka-Yoke
B. SPC
C. FMEA
D. DOE
Q784. Which Lean concept targets overproduction, waiting, and defects as primary waste categories?
A. Kaizen
B. Value Stream Mapping
C. 5S
D. The Seven Wastes (Muda)
Q785. What is the key advantage of using control charts instead of run charts?
A. Provide statistically based decision limits to detect special causes
B. Display correlation strength
C. Summarize data frequency
D. Record categorical counts
Q786. Which Six Sigma tool quantifies financial benefits achieved through process improvements?
A. Cost–benefit analysis
B. SIPOC
C. Pareto chart
D. DOE
Q787. Which visualization technique tracks progress toward multiple key performance indicators (KPIs)?
A. Performance dashboard
B. Fishbone diagram
C. Check sheet
D. Control chart
Q788. Which tool helps teams prioritize improvement actions using weighted criteria scoring?
A. Run chart
B. Pareto chart
C. Flowchart
D. Prioritization matrix
Q789. What does a Cp value less than 1.0 indicate about a process?
A. Process spread exceeds specification tolerance
B. Process mean perfectly centered
C. Process highly capable
D. Measurement error minimal
Q790. Which chart best displays the cumulative percentage of total defects accounted for by each category?
A. Pareto chart
B. Histogram
C. Box plot
D. Scatter diagram

Q791. Which improvement tool uses real-time visual cues to signal process status or abnormal conditions?
A. Andon system
B. Control chart
C. Pareto diagram
D. Fishbone diagram
Q792. Which Lean concept focuses on reducing setup or changeover times to improve flexibility?
A. 5S
B. Kaizen
C. Poka-Yoke
D. SMED
Q793. Which quality improvement method emphasizes rapid, small-scale process changes tested through iterative cycles?
A. PDCA
B. DMAIC
C. Benchmarking
D. Value Stream Mapping
Q794. Which statistical test assesses equality of variances between two samples?
A. F-test
B. t-test
C. Chi-square
D. ANOVA
Q795. Which technique graphically displays workflow steps along with data on time or quantity for each?
A. Process map
B. Swimlane diagram
C. Histogram
D. Scatter plot
Q796. What is the objective of performing capability analysis using Cpk?
A. Determine how centered a process is within specification limits
B. Identify main root causes
C. Measure supplier reliability
D. Predict equipment wear rate
Q797. Which Lean Six Sigma concept visually tracks flow efficiency through work and wait times?
A. Value Stream Map
B. Pareto Chart
C. Control Chart
D. Run Chart
Q798. Which tool quantifies and prioritizes potential design risks before production?
A. Design FMEA
B. SPC chart
C. DOE matrix
D. Benchmark study
Q799. Which graphical tool displays hierarchical relationships among key quality elements or objectives?
A. Flowchart
B. Matrix diagram
C. Fishbone diagram

D. Tree diagram

Q800. Which continuous-improvement approach integrates statistical control with waste reduction to achieve near-perfect performance?

A. Lean Six Sigma
B. Kaizen
C. TQM
D. Benchmarking

Answer key and Explanation (701-800)

Q701. Answer: B
Explanation: The matrix connects CTQs with process factors. Option A – SPC focus. Option C – Evaluation only. Option D – Not its function.
Chapter V – Quality Tools & Techniques
Q702. Answer: B
Explanation: Benchmarking identifies performance gaps via external comparison. Option A – SPC tool. Option C – FMEA task. Option D – Too narrow.
Chapter V – Quality Tools & Techniques
Q703. Answer: A
Explanation: Interaction plots show combined factor effects. Option B – Distribution only. Option C – Rank ordering. Option D – Process flow, not analysis.
Chapter V – Quality Tools & Techniques
Q704. Answer: B
Explanation: A run of seven suggests special cause per Western Electric rules. Option A – Random = alternating. Option C – No shift. Option D – Irrelevant.
Chapter V – Quality Tools & Techniques
Q705. Answer: A
Explanation: FTA models failure logic for hazard ranking. Option B – Defines process scope. Option C – Collects data. Option D – Shows frequency only.
Chapter V – Quality Tools & Techniques
Q706. Answer: B
Explanation: ANOVA assesses differences among multiple means. Option A – Two groups only. Option C – Categorical data. Option D – Variance comparison only.
Chapter V – Quality Tools & Techniques
Q707. Answer: A
Explanation: Gauge R&R quantifies repeatability and reproducibility error. Option B – Monitors process output. Option C – Uses validated data. Option D – Models relations only.
Chapter V – Quality Tools & Techniques
Q708. Answer: B
Explanation: Pareto shows cumulative contribution emphasizing the vital few. Option A – No cumulative view. Option C – Raw counts only. Option D – Shows correlation.
Chapter V – Quality Tools & Techniques
Q709. Answer: B
Explanation: Repeatedly asking “why” drills to underlying cause. Option A – SPC focus. Option C – Categorization. Option D – FMEA function.
Chapter V – Quality Tools & Techniques
Q710. Answer: A
Explanation: Decision trees evaluate expected value and risk trade-offs. Option B – Descriptive. Option C – Monitoring only. Option D – Idea grouping.
Chapter V – Quality Tools & Techniques
Q711. Answer: C
Explanation: Gauge R&R studies separate total measurement variation into repeatability and reproducibility components, clarifying system error sources. Histograms show only frequency distribution, scatter diagrams explore correlation between variables, and control charts detect process shifts rather than measurement system integrity.
Chapter V – Quality Tools & Techniques

Q712. Answer: A

Explanation: The affinity diagram groups related ideas to reveal themes and relationships, promoting organized thinking. Pareto charts rank problem frequency, flowcharts map process steps without exploring idea relationships, and histograms only display data distributions rather than conceptual connections or clustering patterns among brainstormed ideas.

Chapter V – Quality Tools & Techniques

Q713. Answer: B

Explanation: Design of Experiments (DOE) intentionally varies inputs to observe their effects and interactions on outputs, ensuring statistically valid conclusions. ANOVA only tests mean differences, regression assesses correlation rather than controlled causation, and a control plan defines monitoring activities rather than experimenting with variable interactions.

Chapter V – Quality Tools & Techniques

Q714. Answer: A

Explanation: A Gantt chart graphically tracks task schedules and overlaps for effective time management. Flowcharts illustrate process flow but not timing, scatter plots display variable correlations, and Pareto diagrams rank issues by frequency instead of managing project progression or deadline coordination.

Chapter V – Quality Tools & Techniques

Q715. Answer: C

Explanation: The mean represents the arithmetic average and central location in symmetrical distributions. The median marks the middle value unaffected by extreme outliers, the mode indicates the most frequent observation, and the range only measures spread rather than position within the dataset.

Chapter V – Quality Tools & Techniques

Q716. Answer: A

Explanation: Control charts visually separate common from special cause variation, signaling process instability before defects arise. They do not evaluate individual performance, establish specifications, or replace inspection schedules, but rather sustain process predictability through ongoing statistical feedback and rapid anomaly detection.

Chapter V – Quality Tools & Techniques

Q717. Answer: A

Explanation: Flowcharts map process sequences, clarifying where failures originate or controls should be applied. Control plans describe monitoring details but not visualization, run charts track time trends without step context, and histograms reveal frequency distributions not procedural fault locations.

Chapter V – Quality Tools & Techniques

Q718. Answer: B

Explanation: Fault Tree Analysis (FTA) uses logic gates to trace root causes contributing to a top event. Fishbone diagrams categorize causes qualitatively, Pareto charts prioritize issues by occurrence, and scatter diagrams explore variable correlations without hierarchical failure logic representation.

Chapter V – Quality Tools & Techniques

Q719. Answer: A

Explanation: Capability analysis compares process spread to specification limits, quantifying ability to meet requirements through indices Cp and Cpk. It does not signal control status (that's SPC's role), assess personnel performance, or replace normality testing required before capability computation.

Chapter V – Quality Tools & Techniques

Q720. Answer: A

Explanation: Flowcharts depict sequential process actions and decision nodes, clarifying workflow logic. Histograms show frequency distributions, control charts track process variation over time, and matrix diagrams present relationships between factors but not operational sequence or decision logic flow.

Chapter V – Quality Tools & Techniques

Q721. Answer: A

Explanation: A prioritization matrix quantifies team evaluations to rank alternatives or problems objectively. Check sheets collect raw data, histograms summarize distributions, and scatter plots analyze correlation, not prioritization. This structured matrix helps allocate improvement resources effectively and align focus with strategic quality objectives.

Chapter V – Quality Tools & Techniques

Q722. Answer: D

Explanation: Decision trees map alternative paths, probabilities, and expected values to aid rational choices under uncertainty. Flowcharts describe sequences without quantitative evaluation, Pareto charts rank categories by frequency, and control charts track variation rather than guide risk-based selection among decision alternatives.

Chapter V – Quality Tools & Techniques

Q723. Answer: A

Explanation: Scatter diagrams reveal potential relationships or trends between two quantitative variables, suggesting correlation strength. Run charts track time-based changes, Pareto charts rank categories, and pie charts illustrate proportions, but none evaluate paired numerical association like scatter plots do.

Chapter V – Quality Tools & Techniques

Q724. Answer: A

Explanation: The cause-and-effect diagram systematically organizes potential variability sources into categories for analysis. Control charts quantify variation after monitoring begins, check sheets gather raw data, and Pareto charts prioritize issues only after causes are known. This tool promotes structured root cause identification.

Chapter V – Quality Tools & Techniques

Q725. Answer: A

Explanation: R^2 indicates how much output variance the independent variables explain, reflecting model fit. P-values test significance, standard error estimates prediction precision, and mean square supports variance analysis but not directly fit evaluation. High R^2 suggests strong predictive reliability.

Chapter V – Quality Tools & Techniques

Q726. Answer: B

Explanation: Attribute data classify outcomes into categories like defective or non-defective, based on counts rather than measurements. Variable data are continuous, nominal data lack order, and ordinal data reflect rank without quantitative intervals. Counting defects is attribute inspection.

Chapter V – Quality Tools & Techniques

Q727. Answer: A

Explanation: Histograms group continuous data into intervals to show frequency distributions and process spread. Control charts plot data over time, Pareto diagrams rank defect categories, and scatter plots depict correlation without frequency bins. Histograms aid distribution interpretation.

Chapter V – Quality Tools & Techniques

Q728. Answer: A

Explanation: SPC uses control charts and statistical rules to differentiate common from special cause variation. DOE tests factors under controlled conditions, reliability analysis estimates lifetime, and benchmarking compares performance externally without statistical monitoring.

Chapter V – Quality Tools & Techniques

Q729. Answer: A

Explanation: Check sheets standardize real-time data collection for accuracy and completeness at the point of activity. They don't rank causes or perform statistical analysis but supply organized input for subsequent tools like Pareto or control charts to enable pattern recognition.

Chapter V – Quality Tools & Techniques

Q730. Answer: A

Explanation: Dashboards combine visual indicators such as traffic-light colors to summarize key performance metrics in real time. Histograms and scatter plots analyze data sets but lack dynamic status representation, while control charts monitor process stability rather than project completion progress.

Chapter V – Quality Tools & Techniques

Q731. Answer: B

Explanation: Gauge R&R isolates measurement variability by quantifying repeatability and reproducibility across instruments and operators. Design of Experiments explores controlled input changes, ANOVA only partitions variance statistically without diagnostic context, and regression predicts relationships but cannot attribute variation to measurement components.

Chapter V – Quality Tools & Techniques

Q732. Answer: A

Explanation: Flowcharts display stepwise actions, decision nodes, and relationships, improving comprehension of process flow and bottlenecks. Pareto charts prioritize categories, fishbone diagrams classify causes, and histograms present numerical frequency distributions, none portraying activity order or procedural decision logic visually like flowcharts.

Chapter V – Quality Tools & Techniques

Q733. Answer: A

Explanation: Pareto charts rank problem categories by cumulative frequency to focus attention on the vital few causes driving most defects. Control charts monitor variation, scatter diagrams explore correlations, and affinity diagrams cluster ideas without quantifying contribution magnitude or cumulative effect.

Chapter V – Quality Tools & Techniques

Q734. Answer: B

Explanation: Cause-and-effect diagrams systematically categorize possible causes into logical groups such as methods, materials, or environment, aiding root-cause brainstorming. Run or control charts depict temporal performance, capability indices measure spread versus limits, and priority matrices allocate resources, not diagnose causes.

Chapter V – Quality Tools & Techniques

Q735. Answer: A

Explanation: Regression analysis calculates correlation coefficients indicating direction and magnitude of variable relationships. ANOVA compares group means, chi-square assesses categorical independence, and histograms illustrate distributions only. Regression quantifies predictive linear strength, guiding improvement through variable-impact understanding.

Chapter V – Quality Tools & Techniques

Q736. Answer: A

Explanation: Attribute data record categorical outcomes such as "acceptable" or "reject," supporting counts rather than continuous measures. Variable data are measured quantities, ordinal imply ranking, and interval maintain equal spacing but lack true zero. Attributes enable proportion defective metrics.

Chapter V – Quality Tools & Techniques

Q737. Answer: B

Explanation: Control charts plot data against statistical limits to reveal small shifts or trends signaling special causes. Run charts omit control limits, Pareto charts rank categories rather than time trends, and histograms lack temporal sequencing, limiting early drift detection capability.

Chapter V – Quality Tools & Techniques

Q738. Answer: B

Explanation: Box-plots summarize data distribution, median, quartiles, and outliers, enabling rapid visual comparison of variability between groups. Pareto or fishbone charts rank causes, flowcharts show process steps, and histograms lack median and outlier visualization precision characteristic of box-plots.
Chapter V – Quality Tools & Techniques

Q739. Answer: A

Explanation: Gauge R&R design assigns repeated trials to various operators and instruments, ensuring balanced measurement representation and reliable error partitioning. Random sampling lacks structured repetition, stratified sampling divides populations for estimation, and control plans govern monitoring rather than measurement-system study design.
Chapter V – Quality Tools & Techniques

Q740. Answer: A

Explanation: Benchmarking evaluates internal performance versus best-in-class organizations to identify improvement opportunities. DOE experiments with factors internally, SPC maintains process stability, and FMEA prioritizes risk severity; benchmarking uniquely drives competitive insight and target setting for excellence.
Chapter V – Quality Tools & Techniques

Q741. Answer: A

Explanation: Frequent oscillations imply unnecessary adjustments introducing extra variability—classic tampering behavior. Seven points one side signal sustained shift, sudden limit breach shows special cause, and downward trend suggests drift; oscillation best reflects over-control interference.
Chapter V – Quality Tools & Techniques

Q742. Answer: A

Explanation: MTBF quantifies expected operational time before failure, serving as a reliability indicator. Cpk and sigma levels measure process capability, while R^2 gauges statistical model fit, not component dependability. Higher MTBF means greater product reliability.
Chapter V – Quality Tools & Techniques

Q743. Answer: D

Explanation: The chi-square test compares categorical data counts to expected distributions, revealing independence or goodness-of-fit. T-tests examine mean differences, F-tests analyze variance ratios, and ANOVA extends F-test to multiple groups but not categorical proportions directly.
Chapter V – Quality Tools & Techniques

Q744. Answer: A

Explanation: Process mapping identifies every input, output, and interaction to reveal inefficiencies and dependencies. Operator accuracy is an individual metric, capability indexes quantify variation fit, and risk priority numbers belong to FMEA; mapping drives workflow clarity and optimization.
Chapter V – Quality Tools & Techniques

Q745. Answer: C

Explanation: Sigma level expresses distance from mean to limit in standard deviation units, indicating capability and defect potential. Cpk and Cp use ratio forms rather than raw deviation count, while Z-score standardizes single observations, not entire process performance.
Chapter V – Quality Tools & Techniques

Q746. Answer: A

Explanation: Nominal group technique collects individual ideas silently, discusses collectively, and votes anonymously, balancing influence. Affinity diagrams categorize ideas after generation, focus groups favor open discussion susceptible to bias, and fishbone analysis organizes causes not votes.
Chapter V – Quality Tools & Techniques

Q747. Answer: A

Explanation: Two of three points within two sigma of a limit suggest systematic shift per Western Electric rules. Alternation implies randomness, central points indicate stability, and tight clustering near mean shows reduced variation not shift.
Chapter V – Quality Tools & Techniques
Q748. Answer: A
Explanation: Building a Pareto chart begins with accurate category frequency data to rank from highest to lowest impact. Capability indices and control limits belong to SPC, while Ishikawa diagrams identify causes, not quantify their frequency for prioritization.
Chapter V – Quality Tools & Techniques
Q749. Answer: D
Explanation: Weibull plots linearize failure distributions to estimate shape and scale parameters, revealing device life characteristics. Run charts track sequence only, histograms show frequency without time dimension, and control charts monitor process variation not product life.
Chapter V – Quality Tools & Techniques
Q750. Answer: A
Explanation: Failure Mode and Effects Analysis (FMEA) calculates Risk Priority Numbers by multiplying severity, occurrence, and detection, ranking issues for prevention. SPC controls ongoing variation, benchmarking compares performance, and DOE tests factors experimentally rather than prioritizing risk.
Chapter V – Quality Tools & Techniques
Q751. Answer: A
Explanation: Regression analysis quantifies how one variable predicts another, providing both correlation strength and direction. ANOVA compares mean differences among groups, chi-square tests categorical data independence, and control charts monitor process variation rather than measuring variable correlation quantitatively.
Chapter V – Quality Tools & Techniques
Q752. Answer: A
Explanation: Fishbone diagrams organize causes into structured branches such as people, methods, and equipment to locate root contributors. Pareto charts rank categories by impact, histograms show data frequency, and flowcharts visualize process flow, not causal structure of quality problems.
Chapter V – Quality Tools & Techniques
Q753. Answer: A
Explanation: A control plan details monitoring metrics, control methods, and reaction plans to maintain process consistency after improvement. It does not schedule projects, rank issues, or assess vendors but ensures ongoing product conformity through structured process control documentation.
Chapter V – Quality Tools & Techniques
Q754. Answer: D
Explanation: Check sheets standardize data capture, promoting uniform documentation of occurrences or defect types at the source. Flowcharts depict processes, Pareto charts summarize counts post-collection, and control charts analyze variation trends rather than collecting observational data directly.
Chapter V – Quality Tools & Techniques
Q755. Answer: A
Explanation: SPC distinguishes random variation from assignable causes using control charts, enabling timely correction before defects occur. It does not perform FMEA ranking, supplier benchmarking, or satisfaction assessment but maintains production stability through continuous data-driven control.
Chapter V – Quality Tools & Techniques
Q756. Answer: A
Explanation: Matrix diagrams cross-reference categories to reveal relationships or dependencies among factors. Histograms illustrate distributions, run charts track time trends, and scatter plots correlate

numerical pairs. Matrices clarify complex interdependencies, supporting prioritization and cause linkage analysis effectively.

Chapter V – Quality Tools & Techniques

Q757. Answer: A

Explanation: A high RPN, derived from severity, occurrence, and detection, signifies elevated failure risk requiring prompt mitigation. Low occurrence lowers RPN, strong control reduces detection risk, and acceptable risk corresponds to lower scores, not higher, prompting less urgency.

Chapter V – Quality Tools & Techniques

Q758. Answer: A

Explanation: P-charts monitor proportion defective in samples of varying size, ideal for attribute data like pass/fail. C-charts handle count-based defects per unit, $\bar{X}$-R charts measure continuous data, and run charts lack statistical limits to evaluate process stability rigorously.

Chapter V – Quality Tools & Techniques

Q759. Answer: D

Explanation: Defining the problem establishes scope and clarity, ensuring subsequent data and brainstorming focus on the true issue. Acting prematurely or collecting data without context risks wasted effort, while brainstorming follows once the problem is precisely stated.

Chapter V – Quality Tools & Techniques

Q760. Answer: A

Explanation: Six Sigma employs Define, Measure, Analyze, Improve, and Control to reduce variation systematically. Lean targets waste elimination, ISO 9001 defines system requirements, and TQM encompasses cultural quality focus; DMAIC uniquely belongs to Six Sigma's statistical optimization framework.

Chapter V – Quality Tools & Techniques

Q761. Answer: A

Explanation: Control charts visualize process behavior pre- and post-improvement, confirming stability restoration through decreased variation. Pareto diagrams rank categories, flowcharts map processes, and check sheets collect data but cannot statistically confirm variability reduction trends.

Chapter V – Quality Tools & Techniques

Q762. Answer: A

Explanation: Cp and Cpk quantify process potential and centering relative to specifications, guiding performance capability assessment. RPN evaluates failure risks, ANOVA tests group means, and F-tests analyze variance ratios unrelated to specification conformance.

Chapter V – Quality Tools & Techniques

Q763. Answer: D

Explanation: Scatter diagrams expose potential variable correlations, suggesting where adjustments could improve outcomes. Control charts determine stability, inspection intervals are procedural, and control limits arise from statistical analysis—not correlation visualization—making scatter plots ideal for relationship exploration.

Chapter V – Quality Tools & Techniques

Q764. Answer: A

Explanation: Value Stream Mapping visually traces material and information flow to reveal waste and streamline production. Pareto prioritizes frequency, ANOVA analyzes statistics, and cause-and-effect diagrams categorize causes but do not directly evaluate wasteful steps or process flow efficiency.

Chapter V – Quality Tools & Techniques

Q765. Answer: A

Explanation: C-charts track defect counts per inspection unit under fixed sample conditions, ideal for discrete attribute data. P-charts handle varying sample sizes, $\bar{X}$ charts monitor continuous variable means, and scatter plots assess variable relationships, not defect frequency patterns.
Chapter V – Quality Tools & Techniques

Q766. Answer: A

Explanation: 5S—Sort, Set in order, Shine, Standardize, Sustain—enhances efficiency through workplace organization and discipline. It's not a diagnostic or measurement tool but foundational for stable, visual management and continuous improvement.
Chapter V – Quality Tools & Techniques

Q767. Answer: D

Explanation: Impact-effort matrices help teams select improvements offering maximum return for minimal effort. Control charts monitor stability, histograms show data distribution, and FMEA assesses risks; only this matrix optimizes action selection efficiency visually.
Chapter V – Quality Tools & Techniques

Q768. Answer: A

Explanation: Run charts plot sequential data to identify temporal patterns, trends, or shifts signaling process changes. Capability indices quantify fit to specs, Pareto charts rank problems, and fishbone diagrams identify causes, not time-based variation.
Chapter V – Quality Tools & Techniques

Q769. Answer: A

Explanation: Standard deviation quantifies dispersion, indicating variation magnitude from the mean. The mean represents central tendency, median defines midpoint, and range gives only extreme difference, lacking sensitivity to overall variability pattern.
Chapter V – Quality Tools & Techniques

Q770. Answer: A

Explanation: Gemba walks require managers to visit the work area, engage staff, and observe operations firsthand to detect improvement opportunities. Control charts monitor data, Pareto ranks causes statistically, and flowcharts document process logic, not real-time observation.
Chapter V – Quality Tools & Techniques

Q771. Answer: D

Explanation: A repeatability study examines variation when the same operator measures the same part using the same equipment, ensuring measurement consistency. Control charts track process performance, Pareto diagrams prioritize categories, and scatter plots display variable correlations, not measurement reliability.
Chapter V – Quality Tools & Techniques

Q772. Answer: A

Explanation: Fault Tree Analysis (FTA) uses logic gates to map potential failure paths and combinations contributing to a top-level failure. Histograms display frequency, run charts show time-based data, and check sheets capture raw counts without structural fault logic.
Chapter V – Quality Tools & Techniques

Q773. Answer: A

Explanation: The cause-and-effect matrix links process factors to customer requirements, scoring impact strength to focus on key variables. Control limits belong to SPC, supplier metrics to procurement, and capability indices measure variation relative to specifications, not input-output correlation.
Chapter V – Quality Tools & Techniques

Q774. Answer: A

Explanation: Lean emphasizes eliminating non–value-added activities to enhance flow and productivity. Six Sigma targets variation reduction, FMEA ranks risk, and benchmarking compares performance. Lean uniquely streamlines processes by eliminating defects, delays, overproduction, and unnecessary motion.
Chapter V – Quality Tools & Techniques

Q775. Answer: D

Explanation: MSA quantifies measurement variation sources, verifying that data reflect true product characteristics. Supplier reliability and satisfaction trends are business metrics, while bottlenecks involve workflow, not measurement. MSA ensures data credibility before using them for decision-making.
Chapter V – Quality Tools & Techniques

Q776. Answer: A

Explanation: U-charts track average defects per unit with variable sample sizes, accommodating non-constant inspection counts. C-charts assume equal sample sizes, p-charts handle proportion defective, and $\bar{X}$-R charts evaluate continuous data, not defect counts.
Chapter V – Quality Tools & Techniques

Q777. Answer: A

Explanation: Control charts use statistically derived limits to distinguish normal variation from assignable causes. Histograms summarize distribution only, check sheets collect raw data, and Pareto charts rank defect categories without identifying variation sources.
Chapter V – Quality Tools & Techniques

Q778. Answer: A

Explanation: Weibull analysis models time-to-failure behavior, identifying reliability characteristics such as wear-out or early-life failures. DOE examines controlled factors, ANOVA tests mean differences, and benchmarking compares organizations, not product lifetimes.
Chapter V – Quality Tools & Techniques

Q779. Answer: B

Explanation: Creating a histogram begins by gathering and grouping continuous data into classes or bins for visual frequency representation. Root cause analysis and FMEA follow data evaluation, while control limits apply to process control charts, not histograms.
Chapter V – Quality Tools & Techniques

Q780. Answer: A

Explanation: Capability histograms overlay specification limits onto process data distribution, illustrating how closely outcomes meet targets. Scatter plots reveal correlations, flowcharts outline steps, and check sheets collect observations, none showing specification alignment graphically.
Chapter V – Quality Tools & Techniques

Q781. Answer: A

Explanation: Ishikawa diagrams organize brainstormed causes into categories for structured root-cause exploration. They don't track tasks, quantify probabilities, or evaluate suppliers but serve as a systematic cause-identification framework during corrective investigations.
Chapter V – Quality Tools & Techniques

Q782. Answer: A

Explanation: $\bar{X}$-R charts monitor mean and range across subgroups, revealing variation and stability for continuous measurements. P- and C-charts handle attribute data, while run charts lack control limits necessary for statistical process control interpretation.
Chapter V – Quality Tools & Techniques

Q783. Answer: A

Explanation: Poka-Yoke, or mistake-proofing, introduces design mechanisms that prevent errors or make them immediately detectable. SPC monitors variation, FMEA assesses risk severity, and DOE explores factor influence—none focus specifically on prevention by design.

Chapter V – Quality Tools & Techniques

Q784. Answer: D

Explanation: The Seven Wastes define overproduction, waiting, transport, excess processing, inventory, motion, and defects as efficiency losses. Value Stream Mapping visualizes flow, 5S organizes workspaces, and Kaizen promotes continual improvement; Muda classifies specific waste sources.

Chapter V – Quality Tools & Techniques

Q785. Answer: A

Explanation: Control charts apply calculated upper and lower limits to identify special-cause variation statistically, enabling early corrective action. Scatter plots reveal correlations, histograms summarize frequencies, and check sheets collect counts, not monitor control statistically.

Chapter V – Quality Tools & Techniques

Q786. Answer: A

Explanation: Cost–benefit analysis compares improvement costs against savings to determine project viability and success. SIPOC maps process boundaries, Pareto charts prioritize issues, and DOE evaluates variable impacts, but none measure economic return directly.

Chapter V – Quality Tools & Techniques

Q787. Answer: A

Explanation: Dashboards integrate KPIs into visual panels summarizing performance in real time for management review. Fishbone diagrams identify causes, check sheets gather raw data, and control charts focus on individual process metrics rather than broad indicator tracking.

Chapter V – Quality Tools & Techniques

Q788. Answer: D

Explanation: Prioritization matrices assign numerical weights to evaluation criteria, ranking actions objectively based on total scores. Pareto charts rank frequency data, flowcharts show process sequences, and run charts monitor trends without decision weighting.

Chapter V – Quality Tools & Techniques

Q789. Answer: A

Explanation: Cp below 1.0 means process variation exceeds allowable tolerance, indicating potential nonconformance. Centering affects Cpk, not Cp, high capability implies Cp >1.33, and measurement error isn't measured by this index.

Chapter V – Quality Tools & Techniques

Q790. Answer: A

Explanation: Pareto charts combine bars and cumulative line graphs to show category contribution toward total defects, highlighting key priorities. Histograms display frequency only, box plots depict variability, and scatter diagrams explore correlations, not cumulative proportions.

Chapter V – Quality Tools & Techniques

Q791. Answer: A

Explanation: Andon systems employ lights or audible signals on production floors to immediately alert staff to issues, enabling rapid response. Control charts record data trends, Pareto diagrams963 rank defects afterward, and fishbone diagrams analyze causes retrospectively, not provide live process visibility.

Chapter V – Quality Tools & Techniques

Q792. Answer: D

Explanation: Single-Minute Exchange of Dies (SMED) minimizes changeover time by separating internal from external tasks, enhancing responsiveness. Kaizen drives continuous incremental improvement, Poka-Yoke prevents mistakes, and 5S organizes workplaces but doesn't directly reduce equipment setup durations.

Chapter V – Quality Tools & Techniques

Q793. Answer: A

Explanation: Plan-Do-Check-Act (PDCA) cycles implement incremental experiments, evaluating outcomes before full deployment. DMAIC belongs to Six Sigma, benchmarking compares organizations, and Value Stream Mapping charts workflow; PDCA uniquely promotes fast learning through continuous feedback loops.

Chapter V – Quality Tools & Techniques

Q794. Answer: A

Explanation: The F-test compares variance ratios to evaluate equality of dispersion between two data sets. T-tests compare means, chi-square analyzes categorical frequencies, and ANOVA extends mean comparison to several groups, relying itself on variance ratios already tested by F.

Chapter V – Quality Tools & Techniques

Q795. Answer: B

Explanation: Swimlane diagrams organize process steps by responsible function or department, combining timing or quantity information for clarity. Process maps outline general flow, histograms present distributions, and scatter plots reveal variable relationships, not role-based step ownership.

Chapter V – Quality Tools & Techniques

Q796. Answer: A

Explanation: Cpk evaluates both process centering and spread relative to tolerance limits, indicating potential conformance level. Root-cause analysis, supplier evaluation, and predictive maintenance address different objectives, making Cpk the standard for capability alignment assessment.

Chapter V – Quality Tools & Techniques

Q797. Answer: A

Explanation: Value Stream Mapping documents process steps, showing value-added versus idle time to highlight inefficiencies. Pareto charts rank issues, control charts monitor variation, and run charts track trends; VSM uniquely displays both material and information flow.

Chapter V – Quality Tools & Techniques

Q798. Answer: A

Explanation: Design Failure Mode and Effects Analysis (DFMEA) anticipates product design failures by evaluating severity, occurrence, and detection, assigning risk priority numbers to mitigate issues early. SPC controls process outputs, DOE tests factors, and benchmarking compares external performance, not design risk.

Chapter V – Quality Tools & Techniques

Q799. Answer: D

Explanation: Tree diagrams decompose a broad goal into progressively detailed tasks or causes, clarifying logical structure and dependencies. Matrix diagrams show cross-relationships, fishbones categorize causes of problems, and flowcharts represent sequences but not hierarchical breakdowns.

Chapter V – Quality Tools & Techniques

Q800. Answer: A

Explanation: Lean Six Sigma combines Lean's efficiency focus with Six Sigma's variation control to deliver defect rates below 3.4 per million opportunities. Kaizen pursues small daily improvements, TQM emphasizes culture change, and benchmarking compares performance, not optimize it statistically.

Chapter V – Quality Tools & Techniques

Made in United States
Orlando, FL
04 November 2026

90218349R00114